Breakthrough Discoveries in Astrophysics, Neuroscience, Medicine, and Evolution

© *David Rowland*

Contents

Proof that a Big Bang Never Happened 3

Einstein's Trilogy of Erroneous Theories 21

The Maximum Distance Light Can Travel 31

Neurophysiology Makes the Autistic Brain Different 37

Autistic People Biologically Cannot Feel Emotion 53

Cholesterol is Irrelevant to Coronary Artery Disease 63

Hypothyroidism: Most Underdiagnosed Disorder 71

DNA is a Binary Computer Program 79

About the Author 89

Proof that a Big Bang Never Happened

© **Rowland D.** The Big Bang Never Happened: A Conclusive Argument. *Journal of Physics & Astronomy* 2020;8(2):193.

Abstract

For over 100 years, the prevailing belief has been that the universe was created by a *big bang* singularity. This speculative event is an impossibility that has become a firmly entrenched notion only because of a fundamental scientific error that few have questioned, until now. This paper provides both logical proof and corroborating scientific evidence that the universe could ***not*** have begun from a singularity, that galaxies are ***not*** receding from the Milky Way, and that we are ***not*** on a collision course with Andromeda. Edwin Hubble made faulty assumptions and significant miscalculations. *Big bang theory* presupposes that somehow the universe spontaneously created itself from nothing. This notion defies both physics and logic, the science of thinking and reasoning. Nothing cannot be the cause of something. Aristotle is reputed to have expressed it this way: *"The notion that there could be nothing that preceded something offends reason itself."*

Introduction

For over 100 years, the prevailing belief has been that the universe was created by a *big bang* singularity. Because of both logical and scientific errors, this speculative event could not possibly have happened.

The *big bang* idea has become firmly entrenched because of a fundamental scientific error compounded by faulty assumptions, presumptive reasoning, and miscalculations. When these oversights are corrected, we are left with zero evidence supporting any of the suppositions that (a) the universe began from a singularity, (b) galaxies are receding from each other, or (c) we are on a collision course with Andromeda.

Every variation of *big bang theory* suggests that somehow the universe spontaneously created itself from nothing. This notion defies both physics and logic, the science of thinking and reasoning. Nothing cannot be the cause of something.

The universe is everything that exists. There is nothing existing outside the universe that could possibly bring it into existence. Aristotle is reputed to have expressed it this way: *"The notion that there could be nothing that preceded something offends reason itself."*

Redshift is Attenuation; Doppler is Distortion

In 1915, astronomer Vesto Slipher observed that light from some spiral nebulae is *redshifted*, meaning that its frequency drops toward the red end of the spectrum and its wavelength correspondingly increases. Slipher falsely presumed that this phenomenon is a Doppler effect in which a light source moving away from the observer stretches the wavelength of the light it emits.[1] If Slipher had understood that the true wavelength of sound actually remains constant during the Doppler effect, he would have realized that redshift is an entirely different phenomenon.

Doppler is distortion. Sound consists of uniform longitudinal waves passing through the elastic medium of air at a constant frequency. When its source movies towards you, identical length waves hit your ear more frequently, distorting the perceived sound to a higher frequency. As a sound source moves away from you, identical length waves hit your ear less frequently, distorting the perceived sound to a lower frequency.

Suppose an ambulance heading towards you at 70 km/h emits musical note **A** (frequency 440 Hz, wavelength 0.773 m). Suppose also that the first note you hear as the siren comes into earshot is **Bb** (466 Hz). As the ambulance passes by, you hear the true **A**440. After the siren passes, you hear in the distance **Ab** (415 Hz). ***The wavelength of the sound*** emitted by the siren (0.773 m) ***never changes***. Both the **Bb** and **Ab** are distortions of the true **A**440 sound.

Light waves are transverse and travel at 3.0 x 10^8 m/s through space, where there is no medium to resist their movement. Thus, light waves can neither bunch together (creating the illusion of increasing frequency)

– nor drift apart (creating the illusion of decreasing frequency). Whatever frequency is measured is the actual frequency of light at that point of observation.

Redshift is simply the measurable tendency of light to attenuate. The velocity and energy of light always remain constant. However, over extreme distances the frequency of visible light gradually diminishes towards the red end of the spectrum while its wavelength increases by a corresponding amount.

In redshift there is **an actual increase in wavelength**. In Doppler, there is only **the illusion of a change in wavelength.** Redshift and Doppler are fundamentally different. To presume they are the same *Doppler-redshift* is rather like referring to a line in geometry as a straight-curve.

For over a century, astrophysicists have been falsely presuming that redshift measures the velocity of a light source away from the observer. Redshift, however, is a function of only two variables, surface temperature and distance, neither of which have anything to do with velocity.

Because the surface temperature of the Sun is $5,500^0$ C, it emits light in the yellow range of the spectrum. Similarly, a star with a surface temperature of $12,000^0$ C emits light at the blue end of the spectrum, and one with a surface temperature of $3,000^0$ C emits light at the red end of the spectrum.

If Star *X* at a temperature of $7,000^0$ C and Star *Y* at $12,000^0$ C are the same distance from Earth, we could simultaneously be receiving light from *X* in the red end of the spectrum and light from *Y* in the blue end of the spectrum. The temptation is to conclude that light from *X* is redshifted and light from *Y* is blueshifted, but that would be a mistake. The light from both *X* and *Y* is being attenuated (redshifted) at the same rate. It is only because light from *Y* started out at a much higher frequency that it has not yet dropped into the red end of the spectrum.

Expansion Theory

In 1925, mathematician Alexander Friedmann proposed that the universe could be either expanding, contracting, or remaining static. He developed equations to predict either the rate of expansion or rate of contraction, once it was known which was the case.

In 1927, astronomer Georges LeMaître independently developed the same equations as Friedmann. LeMaître, however, presupposed that the universe is expanding and provided mathematics to support his foregone conclusion.

In 1929, Edwin Hubble formulated Hubble's law, which states that objects in deep space have a presumed relative velocity away from Earth and their velocity of recession is approximately proportional to their distance from Earth. Hubble's law is considered the first observational basis for expanding universe theory and today is one of the pieces of evidence most often cited in support of the alleged *big bang*.[4]

In 1931, Georges LeMaître published the English version of his earlier paper entitled, "*A homogeneous Universe of constant mass and growing radius accounting for the radial velocity of extragalactic nebulae.*"[5] He initially called his theory the "hypothesis of the primeval atom" and described it as the "cosmic Egg exploding at the moment of creation." In addition to being an astronomer, LeMaitre was also a Catholic priest who felt comfortable with the notion that God had created the atom/egg that subsequently blew up to create the universe. Thus, what later become known as *big bang* theory may have its origin in metaphysics rather than astrophysics.

Circular Reasoning

Every version of expansion theory inadvertently includes its conclusion in its assumption, then uses this assumption to prove its foregone conclusion. This is the logical fallacy of circular reasoning.

In 1912, Henrietta Swan Leavitt discovered a direct relation between the brightness of Cepheid variable stars and the period of their pulsations.[6] This brightness-periodicity relationship tells us at what stage each

Cepheid may be in its unique life cycle – and absolutely nothing about where said star may be located.

Edwin Hubble made three *a priori* assumptions: (1) the universe began at a single point in time; (2) all Cepheids are the same age; and (3) the brightness of Cepheids is a function of their distance. Hubble's circular reasoning is that he assumed all Cepheid stars are retreating from us, then misused Leavitt brightness-periodicity calculations as evidence to show how far Cepheids have travelled.

Both LeMaitre and Hubble calculated what they believed to be radial velocities of nebulae. They did so by taking the supposed velocity they claim to have measured on the vector between Earth and each nebula in question, then using trigonometry to estimate what the velocity would be on a vector from the universe's presumed origin – without having the foggiest idea where said origin could possibly be located. Both scientists started with the *a priori* assumption that the universe was created by a singularity that happened at a specific point in space, then developed calculations to justify their foregone conclusion.

Hubble's "Law"

Hubble's law is fatally flawed – because of statistical anomalies, faulty assumptions, circular reasoning, and data that may have been contrived.

Statistical Insignificance: Edwin Hubble studied 24 galaxies and selected the results from five of these that demonstrated a perfect straight-line relationship between distance and velocity. Five is a statistically insignificant sample size from which to project meaningful data about the entire universe.

Selection Bias: Hubble used only the data of galaxies from which light was redshifted and ignored data of galaxies from which he knew light appeared to be blueshifted (e.g., Andromeda, M86, M90, M98). He thus chose only data that supported his foregone conclusion and ignored data that conflicted with it. This selection bias disqualifies the Hubble theory as constituting a *law* . A law in physics permits no exceptions. Newton's universal law of gravitation, for example, does not allow for the occasional exception whereby some objects fall upwards or repel each other.

Faulty Assumptions: Hubble did not and could not measure velocities of galaxies. Instead, he relied on the following false or unwarranted assumptions to infer velocity:

1. **All galaxies are approximately the same size**. This assumption caused Hubble to overestimate the distances of small galaxies and underestimate the distances of large ones.
2. **The brightness of a Cepheid star is a function of its distance**. The pulsations of these super massive stars are caused by physical changes that are a function of the life cycle of that star, regardless of how far away it may be. An older, brighter Cepheid star with slower pulsations in a nearby galaxy would thus appear to Hubble to be closer than a newer, less bright Cepheid star.
3. **The dimness of a galaxy is a function of its motion away**, i.e., that as a galaxy retreats, its brightness diminishes. Without also measuring the surface brightness of a galaxy (per unit area), we can conclude absolutely nothing about its supposed motion. Only if the surface brightness of a distant galaxy is significantly less than the surface brightness of nearby galaxies is it reasonable to infer that said galaxy is in motion away from us.
4. **The redshifting of light from galaxies is caused by rapid movement of those galaxies away from us.** This error is rampant in mainstream cosmology – that of mistaking redshift for a Doppler effect, whereas they are in fact two fundamentally different phenomena.
5. **The extent of the redshift is proportional to the velocity at which the galaxy is presumed to be retreating**. Again, redshift has nothing to do with any presumed velocity of source.

Fallacy of Presumption (circular reasoning): Hubble inadvertently included his conclusion in his assumption, then used this assumption to prove his conclusion. He (a) presumed that galaxies are accelerating away from us, (b) presumed that redshift measures velocity, then (c) produced estimates of distance to justify that the redshifts in question demonstrated acceleration.

False premise: Hubble based his entire theory on the misconception that redshift measures velocity. Details above make it clear that redshift can only be construed as a measure of distance and temperature of source.

The following table summarizes the estimates from which Edwin Hubble in 1929 concluded that galaxies are receding from the Milky Way at a velocity proportional to their distance.[4] Entries in the "**Distance-EH**" column indicate the distances that Hubble estimated (based on his multiple flawed assumptions).[4] Entries in the "**Presumed Velocity**" column indicate the velocities that Hubble inferred from his measures of redshift (falsely presuming redshift to be a Doppler effect).[4]

Table A: Edwin Hubble's Estimates of Distances and Velocities

Cluster Galaxy	Distance-EH[4] (ly)	Velocity[4] (km/s)	Ratio (Velocity/Distance)
Virgo	78	1,200	15.4
Ursa Major	1,000	15,000	15.0
Corona Borealis	1,400	22,000	15.7
Bootes	2,500	39,000	15.6
Hydra	3,960	61,000	15.4
Average			15.4

The results in the *Ratio* column above are the five points that Hubble posted on a graph to create a remarkably tight straight-line relationship between the distance of a galaxy and how fast it is supposedly moving away. These calculations support a distance-velocity relationship that is considered the ultimate definitive evidence supporting expansion theory.

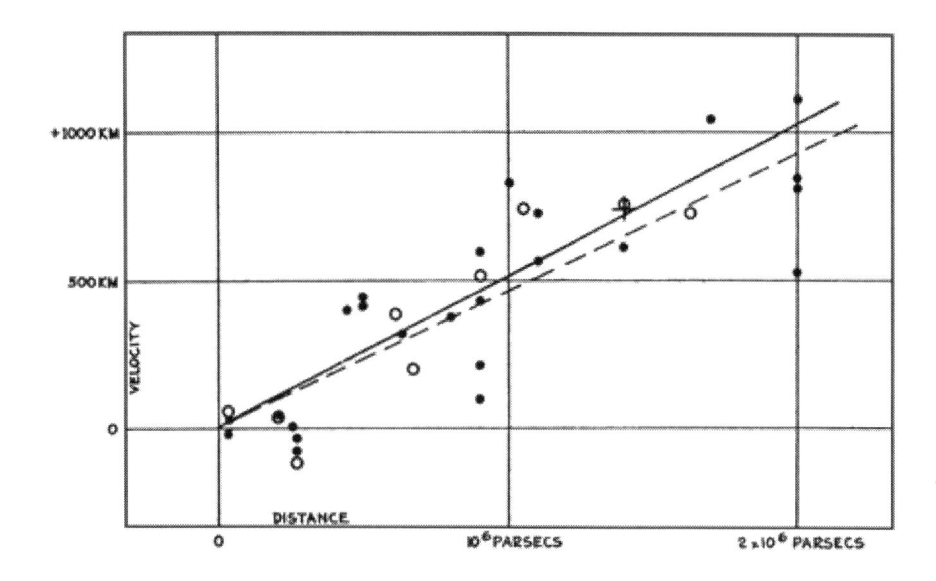

Something is seriously wrong with Hubble's estimates of distance, however. If we substitute modern estimates of distance in the *Distance-Modern* column below, a very different picture emerges. Data in the *Distance-Hubble* column are the figures published by Edwin Hubble in his seminal 1929 paper.[4] Data in the *Distance-Modern* column are published data sourced from the Hipparcos Catalogue of 188 218. On the assumption that the Hipparcos data may be accurate to plus or minus 10%, the estimated *Error Factor* reveals a spread of 22% in each case.

Table B: Modern Estimates of Distance Compared to Edwin Hubble's Estimates

Brightest Star	Distance-Modern (ly)	Distance-Hubble[4] (ly)	Error Factor
Spica (Virgo)[8]	262.19	78	-3.4x
Alioth (Ursa Major)[9]	80.93	1,000	12.4x
Alphecca (Corona Borealis)[10]	75.05	1,400	18.6x
Arcturus (Bootes)[11]	36.72	2,500	68.1x
Alphard (Hydra)[12]	180.30	3,960	22.0x

Edwin Hubble apparently estimated Virgo to be about 3.4 times closer than it really is, and the other star clusters to be from 12.4 to 68.1 times further away than they really are.

If Hubble had used realistic estimates of distance, there would have been no straight line on his graph, only random points indicating a zero correlation between distance and velocity. Thus, it appears that Hubble may have manipulated data to produce the results he wanted.

Either galaxies are moving apart, or they are not. The theory which suggests that the distances between galaxies are increasing is fatally flawed. Therefore, we must presume that galaxies are in the same positions relative to each other that they have always been in. This burden of proof is the same as required in a court of law. If the prosecutor's theory that the defendant is guilty cannot be substantiated, then he must be presumed to be not guilty. The Hubble theory that galaxies are moving apart cannot be substantiated; therefore, we must presume that they are not moving apart.

Hubbles' "law" is thus an interesting mathematical diversion that bears no relation to reality. Redshift is *not* Doppler. Galaxies are *not* retreating from the Milky Way. If galaxies are not in retreat, then their imagined velocity of retreat cannot be increasing.

The Tolman Surface Brightness Test

We now have direct evidence that the universe is *not* expanding. Edwin Hubble's estimates of velocity did not include measurements of surface brightness (i.e., brightness per unit area) of galaxies. Such measurements tell a very different story.

In 1930, mathematical physicist Richard Tolman devised a surface brightness test to determine whether the universe is static or expanding. Tolman's test compares the surface brightness of galaxies to their degree of redshift (measured as z). Tolman believed redshift to be the degree of reduction in energy of each photon.[2]

In a static universe, the light received from an object drops in proportion to the square of its distance, and the apparent area of the object also drops in proportion to the square of its distance, so the surface brightness (light received per surface area) would be constant, independent of distance. In an expanding universe, the surface brightness would decrease with the fourth power of $(1 + z)$.

For 90 years, mainstream astrophysicists have never checked the validity of their assumptions by means of the Tolman test. They all accept on blind faith Slipher's error of mistaking redshift for Doppler.

The Tolman Test Applied

In 2014, Eric Lerner and a team of astrophysicists applied the Tolman test by measuring the surface brightness (per unit area) of over 1,000 near and far galaxies. If galaxies were moving away from each other, they would appear fainter the farther away they get, i.e., their surface brightness would diminish. Lerner's team, however, found that in every case surface brightness remains constant regardless of distance. If any faraway galaxy had been in motion away from us, its surface brightness would have been much less than that of nearby galaxies, a phenomenon that has never been observed. Thus, there is zero tangible evidence that galaxies are moving apart and overwhelming evidence that they are not.[3]

One thousand galaxies in the above study is a statistically significant sample size from which to project meaningful data about the entire known universe. It is 200 times the number of galaxies that Edwin Hubble included in his biased sample.

Conclusion: galaxies are *not* moving apart. They are in the same relative positions to each other that they have always been in.

Andromeda is No Exception

In 1915, Vesto Slipher presumed that galaxies from which light is redshifted are in motion away from us and conversely, those from which light is blueshifted are in motion toward us. Slipher estimated that some galaxies were retreating from us at the rate of 1,100 km/s – and Andromeda appeared to be approaching us at 300 km/s, based on the degree to which its light appeared to be shifted toward the blue end of the spectrum.[1]

In 1924, Edwin Hubble studied Andromeda and estimated that it was 0.9×10^6 ly away from us. (NASA's estimate places Andromeda at about 2.5×10^6 ly away.)

In 1927, Edwin Hubble conveniently omitted the supposedly approaching Andromeda from the data on which he based his conclusion that galaxies are retreating from us at a velocity proportional to distance away (Hubble's "law"). This omission is an example of selection bias at its worst. To include Andromeda would have been like Isaac Newton saying that there are exceptions whereby some kinds of fruit fall upwards.

In 2014, Eric Lerner demonstrated that the surface brightness of 1,000 near and far galaxies is constant, without exception. This observation means that (a) galaxies from which light is redshifted are *not* moving away from us, and (b) galaxies from which light is blueshifted (e.g., M86, M90, M98, and M31/Andromeda) similarly are *not* moving towards us.

If Andromeda were approaching us, its surface brightness (per unit area) would be more intense than the surface brightness of galaxies that are much farther away. Said phenomenon has never been observed. Surface brightness of all galaxies is constant, regardless of their distance away. We are *not* on a collision course with Andromeda.

Blueshift Anomalies

Light emitted by stars and galaxies is subject to redshift attenuation over extreme distances, regardless of its frequency at source. Supernovae emit gamma radiation and high frequency visible light at the blue/violet end of the spectrum which, by the time it reaches Earth, has a lower frequency but is still in the blue end of the spectrum. This gives the false impression that light from supernovae has been blueshifted, but it is in fact heading towards the red end of the spectrum and still has a long way to go to get there.

Those who mistake redshift for motion away also mistake blueshift for motion towards, creating the false impression that supernovae and/or their emissions are heading towards us. Supernovae SN1885A and SN1986J (in Andromeda), SN1994D and SN2007bi (in Virgo), and SN1987A (in the Large Magellan Cloud) emit intense blue and violet light that by the time it reaches us has been redshifted from the very high frequency at which it was emitted at source but still appears to us to be in the blue range of the spectrum.

The presumptive error that redshift/blueshift indicates motion depends on the unwarranted assumption that light from stars is always emitted at or near the middle of the visible light spectrum. Evidence from closer to home reveals that this is not necessarily so. Light from the following nebula in the 700 to 5,000 light-year range is predominantly blue at source: Helix NGC7293, Iris NGC7023, and Swan's Crescent NGC6888.

Light from binary star systems regularly alternates between redshift and blueshift. Examples of such binary systems include Alpha Centauri, Sirius, Beta Lyrae, 61 Cygni, Procyon, 55 Cancri, Castor, and Algol – all of which lie within a distance range of 8 to 90 ly. When these binary stars are at their farthest distance from each other, we experience their light as having been redshifted. When each pair of stars is lined up one behind the other, we observe their light as being in the blue range of the spectrum. This phenomenon suggests that lined up stars together generate more intense heat than either does separately, thus synergistically raising the frequency of emission of their combined light to much higher than either star emits independently of the other

Light from the Virgo cluster is redshifted, but light from five dwarf galaxies within Virgo appears to be blueshifted, including NGC4419, M98, M86, IC3258, and M90. These dwarf galaxies range in distance from 30 to 60×10^6 ly. Classic interpretation of these measurements suggests that the entire Virgo cluster is accelerating away from us whereas five sub-galaxies within Virgo are simultaneously accelerating toward us. This interpretation challenges logic. A more reasonable explanation is that light from these dwarf galaxies is emitted at higher frequencies than is light from the other 2,000 or so galaxies in Virgo.

Only a tiny percentage of known galaxies emit light that appears to have been blueshifted, and the farthest of these is M90, at 60×10^6 ly. One hundred percent of galaxies between this distance and 13×10^9 ly emit light that is redshifted. These two facts strongly suggest that (a) redshift is the natural order of things, and (b) there are no exceptions. Light emitted from every galaxy is always redshifted over extreme distances. If we intercept very high frequency visible light at relatively short distances (e.g., less than 60×10^6 ly), it will have been redshifted from source but could still be in the blue end of the spectrum at our point of observation, thus creating the illusion of a blueshift. We need to let go of the presumption that all galaxies emit light at or near the middle of the visible spectrum.

Cosmic Microwave Background

In 1964, cosmic microwave background (CMB) radiation was discovered by radio astronomers Robert Wilson and Arno Penzias. They heard the CMB as an odd buzzing sound coming from every part of the sky at all times. *Big bang* proponents had been searching for confirming evidence for their singularity theory, and this discovery appeared to be it.

CMB radiation can be detected by telescope in every direction as a patchy background, about 13.4×10^9 ly away. This observation is mistakenly believed to be thermal radiation left over from *recombination*, the epoch during which charged electrons and protons supposedly first became bound to form electrically neutral hydrogen atoms, shortly after the alleged *big bang*. The assumption is that hydrogen, the lightest element, was made exclusively during the *big bang* and in the general area of its supposed origin. However, ionized hydrogen gas in fact permeates the entire universe.

From 1989 until 1993, COBE satellite Explorer 66 investigated the cosmic microwave background. Astrophysicists expected to see evidence of directional dependency (anisotropy) that could be traced back to the site of the alleged *big bang*. That was not what they saw, however. Instead, Explorer 66 measured an isotropic blackbody spectrum with little variation across the sky.[7]

Table C: Blackbody Measurements of Cosmic Microwave Background

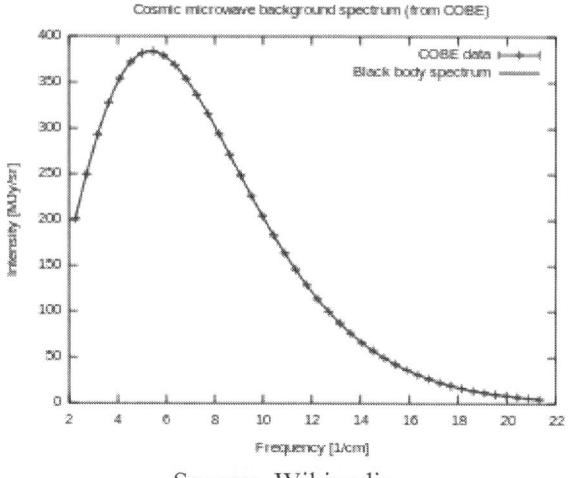

Source: Wikipedia

The above graph represents the cosmic microwave background spectrum as measured by the FIRAS instrument on the COBE. As it turns out, this is the most precisely measured blackbody spectrum in nature. The error bars are too small to be seen even in an enlarged image, and it is impossible to distinguish the observed data from the theoretical curve.

NASA thus confirms that the CMB follows the precise curve for blackbody radiation. A blackbody is an opaque object in space that absorbs radiation of all wavelengths that falls on it. Then, when the blackbody is at a very hot and uniform temperature, it emits its own radiation that is outside the visible spectrum of light. NASA's measurements show that this blackbody curve peaks at 0.3 cm. wavelength and 100 GHz frequency, which is at the high end of the microwave spectrum. The blackbodies in question could simply be interstellar dust.

The cosmic microwave background is smooth and looks the same in all directions for the same reason that a fog looks smooth and uniform in all directions. The CMB thus appears as an electromagnetic fog on optical telescopes and as a static hum on radio telescopes.

Bang Goes the Theory

The prevailing firmly entrenched cosmological model for the universe is that it was created by a *big bang* explosion/singularity that happened some 13.8 billion years ago. This date was arrived at by working backwards in time from equations that purport to measure the universe's rate of expansion.

According to this theory, the entire universe began from some tiny point (or microdot, or quantum) violently exploding out pure energy that almost instantly became particles – and then atoms that eventually combined to form elements, molecules, gases, stars, and galaxies. In other words, the universe spontaneously created itself from nothing.

Proposing a *big bang* or other singularity as cause does not answer the question as to how the universe was created. It simply raises another question as to how the singularity was created.

Points are artificial mathematical abstractions used to specify locations on a graph. Points do not in fact exist. Some variations of the theory are vague about naming what it was that was supposed to have exploded but suggest it was something that had zero dimensions. The same faulty logic prevails: to have zero dimensions is to have zero existence.

Some *big bang* theorists believe that the imagined singularity was a tiny, solid mass with all the matter in the universe compacted into the tiniest bit of space, and then it blew up. Even if it were possible to compress so much mass into such a small space, the intense gravity would have caused it to implode inward rather than explode outward. In addition to this scientific impossibility, there are also two logical errors: (1) all the matter in the universe could not have existed prior to the universe, and (2) something could not have compacted all this matter before any means of compaction existed.

The universe is defined as everything that exists. *Big bang* theory imagines that the something which created the universe existed prior to existence – a contradiction in terms.

Space is defined as the expanse of the universe beyond the Earth's atmosphere. Space is in the universe; the universe is not in space. *Big bang* theory imagines that the something which created the universe was located somewhere before the concept of location (i.e., in space) existed – a second contradiction in terms.

Time is defined as the continuous duration of existence as seen as a series of events. Without existence and events, the concept of time has no meaning. Time is in the universe; the universe is not in time. *Big bang* theory falsely assumes there was a point in time at which time began – a third contradiction in terms.

Many *big bang* proponents claim that it was not a single point in space that exploded but rather every point in the universe participated in the *big bang*. In other words, the explosion happened everywhere at the same time but not at any specific location. Whether one location or every location existed prior to existence is an equally nonsensical argument.

A Child's Perspective

Parent Speaking	Child Responding
Once upon a time, a teeny-weeny dot exploded, creating everything that exists.	Who made this dot?
Nobody, it was just there.	Where? If nothing existed, there was no place to put a dot.
Stop interrupting, I am trying to tell a story.	And how could a dot exist before there was such a thing as existence?
Never mind, it just did.	When did this event happen?
Almost 14 billion years ago.	A year is the time it takes for Earth to circle around the Sun, isn't it?
Yes.	Before there were planets or suns, there was no such thing as years. Correct?
Yes.	So how can you say this story began once upon a time? If there weren't any years, there wasn't any time.
Stop trying to be so logical. Not everything is logical.	Apparently not. So why should I believe this story?
Because I said so.	

Conclusion: A Timeless Universe

Either the universe was created by a (*big bang*) singularity, or it was not. If it was not created at some point in time, then it must be timeless/ageless. There is no third possibility.

There is no need to develop an alternate theory about the origin of the universe. If it did not suddenly pop into existence, then from our frame of reference it must have always been here. The ill-fated *big bang theory* was an attempt to answer *why* there is a universe. Questions of *why*, however, belong to the realm of philosophy rather than science.

References

1. Slipher, Vesto. (1915). "Spectrographic observations of nebulae", *Popular Astronomy*, Vol. 23, pp. 21-24.
2. "Tolman Surface Brightness Test", *Wikipedia*.
3. Lerner, Eric J., Falomo, R, & Scarpa, R. (2014). "UV surface brightness of galaxies from the local universe to z~5", *International Journal of Modern Physics* D, vol. 23, No. 6.
4. Hubble, Edwin. (1929). "A relation between distance and radial velocity among extra-galactic nebulae", *Proceedings of the National Academy of Sciences of the United States of America*, vol. 15, issue 3, pp. 168-73.
5. Lemaitre, Georges. (1927). "A Homogeneous Universe of Constant Mass and Growing Radius Accounting for the Radial Velocity of Extragalactic Nebulae", *Annales Soc.Sci.Bruxelles*, A 47, pp. 49-59,
6. Leavitt, Henrietta S. & Pickering, Edward C. (1912). "Periods of 25 variable stars in the Small Magellanic Cloud", *Harvard College Observatory Circular*, vol. 173, pp. 1-3.
7. "Cosmic Microwave Background", *Wikipedia*: https://en.wikipedia.org/wiki/Cosmic_microwave_background.
8. "Spica (Alpha Virginis, 67 Virginis) Star Facts", https://www.universeguide.com/star/spica.
9. "Alioth (Epsilon Ursae Majoris, 77 Ursae Majoris) Star Facts", https://www.universeguide.com/star/alioth.
10. "Alphecca (Corona Borealis, 5 Coronae Borealis) Star Facts", https://www.universeguide.com/star/alphecca.

11. "Arcturus (Alpha Boötis, 16 Boötis) Star Facts", https://www.universeguide.com/star/arcturus.
12. "Alphard (Alpha Hydrae, 30 Hydrae) Star Facts", https://www.universeguide.com/star/alphard

Einstein's Trilogy of Erroneous Theories

© **Rowland D**. Einstein's Trilogy of Erroneous Theories. *OSP Journal of Physics and Astronomy* 2024;5(1).

Abstract

General Relativity. In 1915, Albert Einstein developed his theory of general relativity, the geometric theory of gravitation that presumes gravity to be the result of geometric distortion of four-dimensional spacetime by massive objects. This alleged distortion supposedly changes the trajectories of objects moving through space and even the paths of light rays as they pass by massive objects. 4-D spacetime is a mathematical illusion that does not exist, does not curve, and cannot possibly interact with the physical force of gravity.

Mass-Energy Equivalence (E = mc²). The *E = mc²* equation in Albert Einstein's theory of special relativity expresses the idea that mass and energy are the same physical entity and can be changed into each other. *E = mc²* is an unverifiable assumption that is considered proof for mass-energy equivalence. This circular reasoning, the logical error of including the conclusion in the assumption then using the assumption to prove the foregone conclusion, invalidates mass-energy equivalence theory. Nuclear fission and nuclear fusion are reactions in which matter is converted to energy. There are no reactions in which energy is converted to matter; it has never happened.

Photon Theory. In 1905, Albert Einstein proposed that light would be better explained by modelling electromagnetic waves as consisting of localized discrete wave-packets, which he called *light quanta*. In 1926, Gilbert N. Lewis coined the term *photon* for this falsely presumed quantum of radiant energy. Individual photons are merely inferred to exist because of their apparent effect on photoelectric systems. This is the logical error of circular reasoning, i.e., including the conclusion in the assumption, then using the assumption to prove the conclusion: it is assumed that photons exist, and measuring their effects is proof of their existence.

Disproof of General Relativity

In 1915, Einstein developed his theory of *general relativity*, the geometric theory of gravitation that is the current description of gravity in modern physics.[1] Einstein proposed that gravity is the result of a geometric distortion of four-dimensional spacetime by massive objects. The more mass that produces gravity in a body, the more distortion you get. This distortion supposedly changes the trajectories of objects moving through space and even the paths of light rays as they pass close by massive objects. Simply stated, massive objects bend the space around them, causing other objects to deviate from the straight lines they otherwise would have followed. Einstein chose the Minkowski spacetime model to depict graphically the gravitational forces presumed by general relativity.[2]

Figure: Hypothetical Fabric of Spacetime

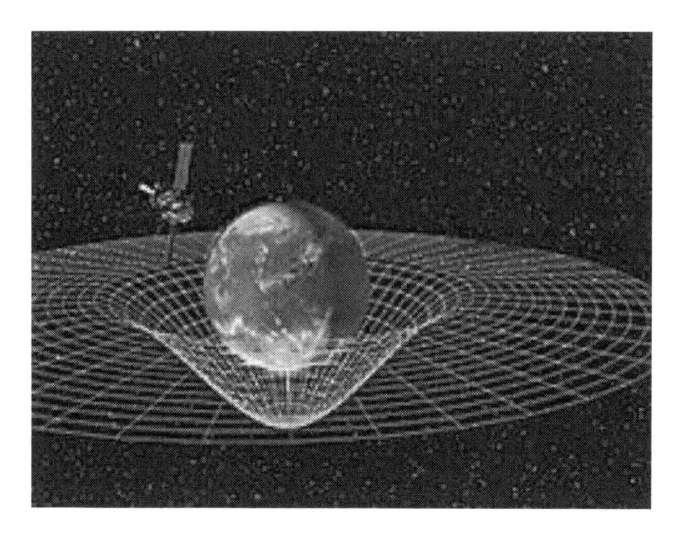

In this model, a massive object (planet or star) appears to be sitting on a fourth-dimensional spacetime fabric, weighing it down, as a heavy ball would do to a rubber membrane in three dimensions. A beam of light passing close by the Sun, for example, would theoretically follow the lip of the curved spacetime fabric, causing it to bend towards the Sun (rather than pass by it in a straight line). General relativity thus depends on the following three unverifiable assumptions: (1) 4-D spacetime is real, (2) spacetime curves, and (3) spacetime interacts with gravitational forces of massive objects.[3]

Spacetime is a mathematical model that supposedly fuses the three dimensions of physical space and the abstract (nonphysical) dimension of time into a single four-dimensional physical continuum. This is a fanciful graphical excursion that bears no relation to reality.

Suppose a world of two dimensions could exist and you wish to represent it on a three-dimensional graph. How would you know if that circle you see is a sphere, a cone, a cylinder, a dome, or something else? It is not possible to extrapolate meaningful information from two dimensions into three, nor from three into four.

Time measures the changing positions of objects and sequences of events that occur within space. Time is thus an abstract (nonphysical) measurement within the 3-D. Time cannot be extracted from space and projected onto a fourth supposedly physical axis with its own independent set of reference points. Whatever model you create that includes mathematical measurements of an intangible dimension cannot possibly be real. To believe in spacetime is to believe in at least one direction to which one cannot point.

Spacetime cannot curve because spacetime is not real. It is an illusion. All Einstein accomplished with 4-D modelling was a fanciful graphic diversion that cannot possibly exist. Nothing about it explains how gravity could possibly bend light.

Although *general relativity* is the accepted definition of gravitation in mainstream physics, this theory is fatally flawed. Spacetime is the geometric illusion that can be expressed algebraically as *3 D + 0 D = 4 D* (where *D* = dimension). Logic tells us that geometric spacetime is not real, does not exist, does not curve, and cannot possibly interact with or be affected by gravity.[3]

Geometry is the mathematics of the properties and relations of points, lines, and surfaces – as well as the relative locations of objects.

Mathematics is an abstract form of measurement and not a physical thing. As such, geometry can neither cause nor be influenced by anything that exists in physical reality. General relativity fails because it presumes that a physical force (gravity) interacts with an abstraction (geometry) that has no physical existence.[3]

Conclusions

Four-dimensional spacetime is a mathematical illusion that is hereby disproven. No theory can be valid if it is based on a false assumption. Therefore, Einstein's theory of General Relativity is also hereby disproven. We are left with the inescapable conclusion that Newton's universal law of gravitation is the only viable explanation for gravity.[4]

Mass-Energy Equivalence ($E = mc^2$) is Invalid

The **$E = mc^2$** equation in Albert Einstein's theory of special relativity expresses the idea that mass and energy are the same physical entity and can be changed into each other. In this equation, the increased relativistic mass (***m***) of a body times the speed of light squared (c^2) is equal to the kinetic energy of that body.[5] Kinetic energy is the form of energy that an object or particle has by reason of its motion.

$E = mc^2$ is an unverifiable assumption that is considered proof for mass-energy equivalence. This is circular reasoning (*aka* begging the question), the logical error of including the conclusion in the assumption, then using the assumption to prove the foregone conclusion. Circular reasoning invalidates the mass-energy equivalence hypothesis.

Nuclear fission and nuclear fusion are reactions in which matter is converted to energy. There are no reactions in which energy is converted to matter; it has never happened. Therefore, mass-energy equivalence is an erroneous theory.

Nuclear fission is a reaction in which the nucleus of an atom splits into two or more smaller nuclei. The fission process releases a very large amount of energy.[6]

In some reactions, matter particles can be destroyed and their associated energy released to the environment as other forms of energy, such as light and heat. One example of such a conversion takes place in elementary particle interactions, where the rest energy is transformed into kinetic energy.[7]

In nuclear weapons, the protons and neutrons in atomic nuclei lose a small amount of their original mass. Nuclear fission allows a tiny fraction of the energy associated with mass to be converted into radiation energy.[8]

Nuclear fusion is the process by which nuclear reactions between light elements form heavier elements. In cases where the interacting nuclei belong to elements with low atomic numbers, substantial amounts of energy are released.

Conclusions

The $E = mc^2$ equation in Albert Einstein's theory of special relativity is an unverifiable assumption that is considered proof for mass-energy equivalence. This circular reasoning, including the conclusion in the assumption then using the assumption to prove the foregone conclusion, invalidates the mass-energy equivalence hypothesis. Nuclear fission and nuclear fusion are reactions in which matter is converted to energy. There are no reactions in which energy is converted to matter; it has never happened. Mass-energy equivalence is an erroneous theory.

Photons are Nonexistent

Light: electromagnetic radiation of any wavelength that travels in a vacuum with a speed of 299,792 meters (186,282 miles) per second.

Photon: an elementary particle that is a quantum of the electromagnetic field, including electromagnetic radiation such as light and radio waves. Photons are massless.

Particle: a small, localized object that can be described by physical properties, such as volume, density, or mass. Particles vary in size or quantity, from subatomic particles like the electron, to microscopic particles like atoms and molecules, to macroscopic particles like powders and granular materials.

Elementary particle: a subatomic particle that is not composed of other particles. The Standard Model lists 61 different elementary particles including electrons, leptons, quarks, fermions, bosons, protons, and neutrons. Photons are excluded from this Standard Model listing.[9]

Something is seriously wrong with the definition of *photon*. Particles are tiny bits of matter that have mass and are localized (i.e., are part of physical objects). Photons are massless and nonlocalized (i.e., radiating everywhere) and thus cannot logically be particles. Photons are not subatomic and thus fall outside the scope of quantum physics.

Visible light is electromagnetic radiation that can be perceived by the human eye. Visible light has wavelengths in the range of 400–700 nanometres (nm), corresponding to frequencies of 750–420 terahertz (THz), between the infrared (with longer wavelengths) and the ultraviolet (with shorter wavelengths).

In 1905, Albert Einstein published a paper in which he proposed that light would be better explained by modelling electromagnetic waves as consisting of localized, discrete wave-packets. He called such a wave-packet a *light quantum*.[10] Einstein thus modified the description of a phenomenon to fit his preconceived notion. Light is ever-present electromagnetic energy that radiates in waves with steady amplitudes and frequencies. Quantum theory is thus irrelevant to the nature of light, which does not propagate in packets. In 1926, physical chemist Gilbert N. Lewis coined the term *photon* for this falsely presumed quantum of radiant energy.[11]

Individual photons are merely inferred to exist because of their apparent effect on photoelectric systems. In a photomultiplier tube, a photon strikes a metal plate and knocks free an electron, initiating an ever-amplifying avalanche of electrons. On a microscopic capacitor, an incident photon generates a charge that can be detected. In a Geiger counter, photons ionize gas molecules.[12] Such inference is fatally flawed, however. What is being observed in all three cases is electromagnetic energy moving electrons. There is nothing in these observations to indicate or even suggest that this electromagnetic energy could be in the form of elementary particles (photons). This is the logical error of circular reasoning, i.e., including the conclusion in the assumption, then using the assumption to prove the conclusion: it is assumed that photons exist, and measuring their effects is proof of their existence.

There is neither physical evidence nor logical reason for the existence of photons. Alleged photon particles are falsely presumed to exist because of faulty logic and misinterpretation of evidence.

In 1804, Thomas Young established the wave theory of light.[13] He did so by means of an interference experiment (predecessor of the double-slit experiment) in which he reflected sunlight with a steering mirror through a small hole and split the beam in half using a paper card. He also mentioned the possibility of passing light through two slits in his description of this experiment.

When light passes through a hole or slit, it diffracts. Diffraction is the interference or bending of waves through an aperture into the region of geometrical shadow of the aperture. The diffracting aperture becomes a secondary source of the propagating wave.

Particles (electrons, protons, atoms) that are fired as projectiles through a double-slit apparatus do not diffract. They are detected as white dots on a screen. Light diffracts. Particles do not. Thus, light cannot be composed of particles.

When particles are allowed to build up one by one before passing through a double slit, however, an artificially induced diffraction pattern emerges.[14] Misinterpretation of these results became the basis of erroneous wave-particle duality theory, namely that quantum entities supposedly exhibit either particle or wave properties depending on the experimental circumstances.

Conclusions

Photon theory is a failed hypothesis. Alleged photon particles have falsely been presumed to exist because of faulty logic and misinterpretation of evidence. Double slit experimental results became the basis of wave-particle duality theory, i.e., that quantum entities supposedly exhibit either particle or wave properties depending on experimental circumstances. Light, however, is not a quantum entity. It is electromagnetic energy that propagates in steady waves. Particles are tiny bits of matter that are incapable of independent motion and thus have no intrinsic wavelike properties. To extract particles from matter and fire them through slits as projectiles is an artificial construct that is irrelevant to the study of light. Light is a continuous electromagnetic wave. Particles are matter. There is no duality.

References

1. Renn J. (ed.) *The Genesis of General Relativity, Vol. 2.* New York, 2007: Springer, pp 819-830.
2. Corry L. Hermann Minkowski and the postulate of relativity. *Arch Hist Exact Sci* 1997;514):273-314
3. Rowland, D. What Einstein did not consider about gravity. *OSP Journal of Physics and Astronomy* 2020;1(1).
4. Rowland, D. Disproof of spacetime and general relativity. *OSP Journal of Physics and Astronomy* 2023;2(1).
5. Arora MG, Singh M. *Nuclear Chemistry.* Delhi, 1994: Anmol Publications, p 202.
6. Bethe HA. *The hydrogen bomb.* Bulletin of the Atomic Scientists 1950;6(4): 99-104.
7. Braibant S, Giacomelli G, Spurio M. *Particles and Fundamental Interactions: An Introduction to Particle Physics 2nd ed.* New York: 2012, Springer, pp 1-3.
8. Braibant S, Giacomelli G, Spurio M. *Particles and Fundamental Interactions: An Introduction to Particle Physics.* New York: 2009, Springer, pp 313-314.
9. Baser PA, Imbert M. *Vision.* Cambridge MA: 1992, MIT Press, p 50.

10. Einstein A. Uber einen die Erzeugung und Verwandlung des Lichtes betreffenden heuristischen Gesichtspunkt. *Annalen der Physik* 1905;(17):132-148.
11. Joos G. *Theoretical Physics*. London: 1951, Blackie and Son Limited, p 679.
12. Kitchin CR. *Astrophysical Techniques*. Boca Raton: 2008, CRC Press.
13. Young T. Bakerian lecture: experiments and calculations relative to physical objects. *Philosophical Transactions of the Royal Society* 1804;(94):1-2.
14. Messiah A. *Quantum Mechanics*. North Holland: 1966, John Wiley & Sons.

The Maximum Distance Light Can Travel

© **Rowland D.** Calculations to Establish How Far Visible Light Travels before Dropping Out of Sight. *OSP Journal of Physics and Astronomy* 2022;3(2).

> ## Abstract
> The purpose of this study is to determine the maximum distance light can travel before it attenuates below the visible frequency range, i.e., drops out of sight. As light travels extreme distances through space, its frequency slowly diminishes (attenuates). We observe this phenomenon as a *redshift*, the tendency of visible light to drop toward the red end of the spectrum. When redshift is properly understood, its measurements enable us to calculate at what distance light continues to attenuate beneath the visible spectrum. Beyond this limiting distance, there are countless billions of galaxies that are invisible to us.

The Redshift Blunder

In 1915, astronomer Vesto Slipher observed that light from some spiral nebulae is redshifted and falsely presumed he was witnessing a light source rapidly moving away from the observer and somehow stretching the wavelength of light it emits.[1] This is an impossibility. Slipher did not understand how light attenuates and mistakenly believed he was witnessing a Doppler effect.[2]

Redshift and Doppler are two fundamentally different phenomena. In redshift there is an actual increase in wavelength. In Doppler, there is only the illusion of a change in wavelength. Redshift is attenuation whereas Doppler is distortion. To presume they are the same Doppler-redshift is rather like referring to a line in geometry as being a straight-curve.[3]

Light waves are transverse (i.e., oscillate perpendicular to their path) and do not require any medium through which to travel. Sound waves are longitudinal (i.e., vibrate parallel to their path) and can only propagate by compression and rarefaction of the medium through which they travel (e.g., air, water, solids). Light travels through outer space. Sound cannot.

If the source of a sound is moving towards you, identical length waves hit your ear more frequently, distorting the perceived sound to a higher frequency. As a sound source moves away from you, identical length waves hit your ear less frequently, distorting the perceived sound to a lower frequency. This is the Doppler effect.[3]

Redshift is Attenuation

Over extreme distances, light attenuates according to $c = \lambda f$
where c = speed of light; λ = wavelength of light; and f = frequency of light wave.

What $c = \lambda f$ tells us is that as the frequency of light drops over extreme distances, its wavelength correspondingly increases. For over a century, astrophysicists have paid more attention to wavelength than to frequency of redshifted light.

The farther light travels, the greater the degree to which its frequency slowly diminishes. We observe this phenomenon as a *redshift*, i.e., the tendency of visible light to drop toward the red end of the spectrum. The farther away a galaxy is, the more its light shifts toward the red end of the spectrum.

If a distant source emits light in the middle of the spectrum, it can be in the red end of the spectrum by the time we receive it. If, however, that source emits light in the blue end of the spectrum, it will have redshifted but could still be in the blue range by the time we receive it. There is no such thing as a "blueshift" whereby wavelengths shorten and frequency increases. All light is redshifted. Light cannot behave in any other way.

Because the surface temperature of the Sun is $5,500°$ C, it emits light in the yellow range of the spectrum. A star with a surface temperature of $12,000°$ C emits light in the blue end of the spectrum, and one with a surface temperature of $3,000°$ C emits light in the red end of the spectrum.

If Star X at a temperature of 7,000°C and Star Y at 12,000°C are the same distance from Earth, we could simultaneously be receiving light from X in the red end of the spectrum and light from Y in the blue end of the spectrum. The temptation is to conclude that light from X is redshifted and light from Y is blueshifted, but that would be a mistake. The light from both X and Y is being attenuated (redshifted) at the same rate. It is only because light from Y started out at a much higher frequency that it has not yet dropped into the red range of the spectrum.

Redshift is a function of two variables only: (1) frequency at source, and (2) distance travelled. If we know the frequency at source, the frequency at our point of observation can tell us how far that light has travelled. This is all that redshift can tell us. Nothing more.

An Infinite Universe

The alleged big bang never happened. That the universe could have begun from any kind of singularity is both logically impossible and scientifically indefensible. There is no point in time at which time began. Time is in the universe; the universe is not in time. The universe is a limitless, endless infinite expanse that is without beginning or ending.[4]

Space is in the universe; the universe is not in space. Space has no shape and no boundaries. Space is an endless expanse within the infinite universe.[4]

Galazy GN-z11

Galazy GN-z11 enables us to estimate rate of attenuation over its distance of 13.39 billion light-years. Light from GN-z11 is dull red, and its frequency is documented by NASA as being in the low red range of the spectrum.[5,6]

The frequency of visible light ranges from a high of 800 THz to a low of 400 THz. What we know is the frequency of light from GN-z11 at our point of observation (low red). What we do not know is the frequency of light from GN-z11 at its source.

Scenario A

Suppose that GN-z11's frequency at source (f_s) is 590 THz (mid spectrum) and its frequency received (f_{obs}) is 410 THz (low red). This would mean that over 13 billion light-years (Gly), frequency from GN-z11 has dropped by 180 THz. This is equivalent to frequency dropping every billion light-years to 0.9811 of the frequency of the previous billion light-years. We can thus express redshift attenuation (R_A) by the following equation in which distance (D) is in incremental units of one billion light-years (Gly).

$$R_A = f_{obs} = f_s (0.9811)^D$$

When its frequency drops below 400 THz, light is no longer visible. It continues at the speed of light but as electromagnetic energy that cannot be seen. This would happen for GN-z11 at 15 Gly

Scenario B

Suppose that GN-z11's frequency at source (f_s) is 790 THz (high blue) and its frequency received (f_{obs}) is 410 THz (low red). This would mean that over 13 billion light-years (Gly), frequency from GN-z11 has dropped by 380 THz. This is equivalent to frequency dropping every billion light-years to .9508 of the frequency of the previous billion light-years. We can thus express redshift attenuation (R_B) by the following equation in which distance (D) is in incremental units of one billion light-years (Gly).

$$R_B = f_{obs} = f_s (0.9508)^D$$

When its frequency drops below 400 THz, light is no longer visible. It continues at the speed of light but as electromagnetic energy that cannot be seen. This would happen for GN-z11 at 14 Gly.

Unseen Galaxies

From the above calculations we can draw two conclusions: (1) The extreme distances that light travels is more significant to its rate of attenuation than is its frequency at source; and (2) The maximum distance that visible light can travel before dropping out of sight is likely to be 15 billion light-years (Gly).

The Hubble Space Telescope creates for us a spherical horizon with a radius of 13.4 billion light-years. We have no way of knowing what lies beyond this horizon. The above analysis suggests that between 13.4 and 15 Gly there may be one or more galaxies visible to us in the low red frequency range (410 THz.). However, beyond 15 Gly no galaxies will be visible because the frequency of the light they emit has dropped below the visible spectrum creating the illusion that we would be looking out at empty space.

It is a convenience of nature that there should be a maximum distance that visible light can travel. Were this not so, the night sky would be ablaze with a patchwork blanket of light rendering us incapable of distinguishing one celestial object from another. We would never be able to understand the cosmos or our place in it.[3,7]

Conclusion

Over extreme distances through space, the energy of light gradually diminishes (attenuates). We observe this phenomenon as a redshift, the tendency for the frequency of light to drop toward the red end of the spectrum. Redshift measurements indicate that the maximum distance light can travel may be 15 billion light-years, at which distance it will have attenuated into a frequency range that is below the visible spectrum. Beyond this 15 Gly limit there are countless billions of galaxies that are invisible to us.

References

1. Slipher V. Spectrographic observations of nebulae. *Popular Astronomy* 1915;(23):21-24.
2. Rowland D. The redshift blunder has been obstructing cosmology for over a century. *OSP Journal of Physics and Astronomy* 2021;2(2).
3. Rowland D. Redefining redshift as attenuation. *OSP Journal of Physics and Astronomy* 2020;1(1)

4. Rowland D. An infinite universe. *OSP Journal of Physics and Astronomy* 2021;2(1).
5. "Telescopes Spy Ultra-Distant Galaxy". NASA.
6. "List of the Most Distant Astronomical Objects". Wikipedia.org.
7. Rowland D. How far visual light can travel. *OSP Journal of Physics and Astronomy* 2021;2(2).

Neurophysiology Makes the Autistic Brain Different

© **Rowland D**. Neurophysiology is What Makes the Autistic Brain Different. *Journal of Neurology, Psychiatry, and Brain Research* 2023;(02).

Abstract

About 70% of those believed to be on the autism spectrum may not be autistic. This apparent epidemic of false diagnoses is being created by professionals who diagnose by ticking off symptoms on a checklist without questioning the causes of said symptoms, and without understanding the innate neurophysiology of the autistic brain. A dysfunctional cingulate gyrus (CG) hyperfocuses attention in the left frontal lobe (logical/analytical) with no ability to access the right frontal lobe (emotional/creative), which plays a central role in spontaneity, social behavior, and nonverbal abilities. Autistic people live in a specialized inner space that is entirely intellectual, free from emotional and social distractions. They have no innate biological way of emotionally connecting with other people. Autistic people process their emotions intellectually, a process that can take 24 hours, by which time it is too late to have felt anything. An inactive amygdala makes it impossible for autistic people to experience fear. Because they do not feel emotion, they have no emotional memories. All memories are of events that happened about which they felt no emotion at the time and feel no emotion when talking about it afterward.

Introduction

Definition: Autism is perpetual and unrelenting hyperfocus, the state of intense single-minded concentration fixated on one thing at a time to the exclusion of everything else, including one's own emotions. The probable cause of hyperfocus is a dysfunctional cingulate gyrus (CG), that part of the brain which focuses attention.[1]

Description: Autism is an inherent neurophysiological difference in how the brain processes information. Autistic people live in a specialized inner space that is entirely intellectual, free from emotional and social distractions. They observe the world in detail without feeling any emotional attachment to what they see. [1]

Autism is a neurophysiological idiosyncrasy. The only thing different about an autistic brain is the specialized way in which it processes information. As such, autism does not fit the medical definition of *disorder* (i.e., pathological or diseased condition of mind or body). Mozart, Paganini, Newton, Darwin, Jefferson, Edison, Tesla, and Einstein were autistic and obviously not suffering from any mental pathology.[2]

Historical Research

Autism, from the Greek word meaning self, was coined in 1911 by Swiss psychiatrist, Eugen Bleuler, who used it to describe withdrawal into one's inner world.[3] Autistic children appear to be in a world of their own, isolated, and alone with senses that can easily overload. These children talk endlessly about one subject, engage in repetitive behaviors (e.g., wringing hands, rocking body), continually repeat certain words or phrases (echolalia), and are resistant to change.[4]

In 1943, psychiatrist Leo Kanner studied the case histories of 11 highly intelligent children who shared a common set of symptoms consistent with autism: the need for solitude, the need for sameness, and to be alone in a world that never varied.[5] Kanner assumed that these children came into the world without innate biologically provided ways of emotionally connecting with other people.[6]

In 1944, medical professor Hans Asperger described "a particularly interesting and highly recognizable type of child" who has an autistic personality that is an "extreme variant of male intelligence." Asperger described four boys who had severe difficulties of social integration that were compensated for by the kind of high level of thought or experience that can lead to exceptional achievements in later life. He chose the label autism for this condition as referring to an inherent fundamental disturbance of contact, the shutting off of relations between self and the outside world.[7] Asperger remarked that for those boys, social adaptation has to proceed via the intellect, and in fact they have to learn everything by the intellect. He considered the autistic syndrome to be a stable personality trait that is genetically transmitted in families.[8]

In 1962, psychiatrist Gerhard Bosch compared infantile autism to the Asperger autistic syndrome and considered them to be two variants of the same condition.[9] In the family of the author of this article, one young lad has nonverbal autism and his younger brother has Asperger's, thus confirming that both variations have the same genetic origin.[2]

In 1979, psychiatrist Lorna Wing introduced the term *Asperger syndrome* to describe the autistic personality. Wing personally examined 34 cases fitting Asperger's description of the autism syndrome and found that they had the following 11 traits in common: [10]

- Single-mindedness combined with social isolation,
- Pedantic speech, often consisting of lengthy discourses on favorite subjects,
- Poor comprehension of other people's expressions and gestures,
- Tendency to misinterpret or ignore nonverbal signs,
- Impairment of two-way social interaction,
- Inability to understand rules of social behavior,
- Lack of the intuitive ability to adapt their approaches to fit in with the needs of others,
- Intensely attached to certain possessions,
- Excellent rote memories and intensely interested in one or two subjects,
- Absorb every fact concerning their chosen field and talk about it at length regardless if the listener is interested, and
- Thought processes are confined to a pedantic, literal, and logical chain of reasoning.

In 2020, David Rowland discovered that autism is caused by an inherent neurophysiological idiosyncrasy that creates a state of perpetual hyperfocus, which he defines as intense mental concentration fixated on one thought pattern at a time to the exclusion of everything else, including one's own feelings.[11] Hyperfocus is the sole factor responsible for the autistic person's withdrawal into an inner space that is entirely intellectual. Hyperfocus keeps a person's awareness trapped in the analytical/logical left frontal lobe of the brain with no ability to access whatever may be happening in the right frontal lobe, the place where emotions and social connectivity are felt. Hyperfocus explains all 11 traits of Asperger listed by Lorna Wing above.

The Spectrum Fallacy

Autism does not belong on any alleged spectrum. There is only one autism, and it is 100%. Either you are autistic, or you are not.

In 2013, the American Psychiatric Association merged the following four disorders under the umbrella of autism spectrum disorder (ASD): autism disorder, Asperger syndrome, childhood disintegrative disorder, and pervasive disorder not otherwise specified (PDD-NOS). This alleged spectrum is a basket catch-all for conditions of uncertain similarity.

The American Psychological Association defines autism spectrum disorder (ASD) as any one of a group of disorders typically occurring during the preschool years and characterized by varying but often marked difficulties in communication and social interaction.[12] DSM-5, *the Diagnostic and Statistical Manual of Mental Disorders*, describes autism as being characterized by (1) persistent deficits in social communication and social interaction; and (2) restricted, repetitive patterns of behavior, interests, or activities. These criteria are so vague as to be meaningless. If you do not know what causes certain symptoms, then you know nothing about any presumed disorder in question.

Epidemic of False Diagnoses

In 2018, the Centers for Disease Control (CDC) reported that 1 in 44 children were diagnosed with an autism spectrum disorder, for a prevalence rate of 2.27% of the population.[13] In 2012, a review of global prevalence of autism found 62 cases per 10,000 people, for a prevalence rate of 0.62%.[14] This apparent 266% increase in autism prevalence is in stark contrast to all other disorders in the Diagnostic and

Statistical Manual of Mental Disorders (DSM-5), for which there have been no increase in prevalence over this same 6-year period.[15] These data suggest that 70% of those believed to be on the autism spectrum are not autistic.

A 10-year Swedish study in 2015 concluded that although the prevalence of the autism phenotype has remained stable, clinically diagnosed autism spectrum disorder has increased substantially.[16] Phenotyping is based on observing gene expressions in individuals and relating their conditions to hereditary factors. Nowadays professionals diagnose by ticking off symptoms on a checklist, without questioning the possible causes of said symptoms. This is a major step backward from clinical phenotyping.

A 2016 study reported that many children originally diagnosed with autism spectrum disorder were later found not to be autistic.[17] A comprehensive 2019 study in *JAMA Psychiatry* indicates that autism is being significantly over diagnosed.[18] Dr. Laurent Mottron, co-author of this study, has expressed these concerns: *"The autism category has considerably overextended ... most neurogenetic and child psychiatry disorders that have only a loose resemblance with autism can now be labelled autistic ... you could not have ADHD and autism before 2013, now you can."*[19] Doctors now tend to label as autistic anyone who simply has ADHD and poor socialization.[20]

Neurophysiology of the Autistic Brain

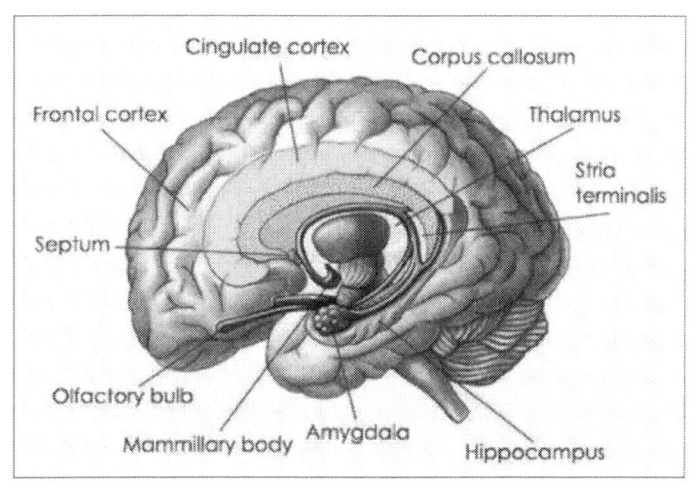

> The neurological structure of the autistic brain is the same as for any other brain. What is different about the autistic brain is how it functions with respect to its neurophysiology.

Table 1: Autistic Neurophysiology

Cingulate Cortex/Gyrus	Dysfunctional	The cingulate gyrus (CG) is that part of the brain which focuses attention. In autism, the CG keeps attention fixated in the left frontal lobe, creating a perpetual state of hyperfocus.
Left Frontal Cortex/Lobe	Dysregulated	In the autistic left frontal lobe, alpha frequencies (8-12 Hz) predominate over beta (12.5-30 Hz), which is the exact opposite of the neurotypical brain. Higher alpha frequencies in the left brain appear to compensate for inability to access creativity and intuition from the right brain.
Right Frontal Cortex/Lobe	Inaccessible	There is normal brainwave activity in the right frontal lobe, with alpha frequencies predominating over beta. However, neural networks may be underdeveloped. The autistic person is completely unaware of anything that happens in the right frontal lobe, the place where emotions and social connectivity are experienced by neurotypical people.
Amygdala	Inactive	The amygdala plays a central role in the expressing of emotions, especially fear. A dysfunctional CG prevents the autistic person from feeling any emotion, with the result that the amygdala is non-functional. An autistic person is incapable of experiencing fear.

In a neurotypical brain, the cingulate gyrus (CG) acts like an automatic transmission that seamlessly switches attention back and forth between frontal lobes, as needed. In autism, a dysfunctional CG keeps the person's attention trapped in the left frontal lobe (logical/analytical) – with no ability to access the right frontal lobe (emotional/creative), which plays a central role in spontaneity, social behavior, and nonverbal abilities. Some neurotypical people are left-brain dominant whereas others are right brain dominant. Autistic people, however, are left brain exclusive. They speak factually, in a monotone voice, and with an expressionless face.[11]

The right frontal lobe, the place where emotions are experienced, is inaccessible to autistic people. The amygdala, the place where emotions are expressed, is inactive in the autistic brain.

These facts are consistent with Leo Kanner's belief that autistic children come into the world without innate biologically provided ways of emotionally connecting with other people.[5]

In a neurotypical brain, the amygdala processes emotions associated with fear and stores emotional memories. When faced with a dangerous situation, the amygdala sounds an alarm that sets off a chain of events: hormones course through the body, pupils dilate, heartrate increases, and the body experiences a "fight or flight" reaction. In extreme situations, all nervous energy goes to the amygdala, which runs totally on instinct and emotion; and that part of the brain that uses logic shuts down completely. In the autistic brain, none of this happens because the amygdala is nonfunctional. In every dangerous situation, the autistic person is fully focused on the event itself and is incapable of feeling fear. Because autistic people do not feel emotion, they have no reaction and no emotional memories. All memories are of events that happened about which they felt no emotion at the time, and about which they feel no emotion when telling someone about it afterward.

Autistic process their emotions intellectually, which process can take 24 hours, by which time it is too late to have felt anything. Physiological anxiety acts as a safety net to warn of any unprocessed emotion.

Hyperfocus also causes various kinds of sensory overload. A sudden loud or high-pitched noise switches hyperfocus to the noise, which the autistic person then experiences with many times the intensity than does a neurotypical person. Seeing too many words on a page may cause cognitive impairment whereby the autistic person's mind goes disturbingly blank. Too many products on shelves and overhearing unwanted conversations in stores may trigger anxiety. Lighting displays can trigger intense anxiety. For some, hyperfocus exaggerates the sense of touch, making close fitting clothing irritating and hugs unbearable.

Autistic Fearlessness

Autistic people have no involuntary fear response. Innate fearlessness makes autistic children oblivious to danger. In life-threatening situations, the autistic adult is fully focused on the event itself and incapable of feeling fear or even nervousness in that moment. She or he feels a mildly heightened sense of awareness while coldly calculating risks and mitigating factors that quickly form an immediate plan of action. The author of this article is autistic and in his entire life, including 17 years of experience in martial arts, has never once felt fear of any kind.[1] He has never had a fight-or-flight reaction and has no awareness of how that could feel.

Sometimes autistic people may intellectualize about fear, for example saying that after thinking about such-and-such decided it could be a scary thing. However, they are incapable of experiencing any actual fear. If you encounter someone who has never felt fear, this person is most probably locked into autistic hyperfocus.[1]

Litmus Test

Hyperfocus is the unique and defining causal state of autism that creates all of its characteristics. Hyperfocus prevents someone from dividing attention between two thought patterns at the same time. An autistic person talking to you is incapable of feeling any emotion in that moment. The surest way to find out if someone is autistic is to ask these five questions, to which you will receive these responses.[1]

1.	How often do you cry?	*"never"* or *"rarely"*
2.	How often do you laugh?	*"never"* or *"rarely"*
3.	What are you afraid of?	*"nothing"* or an intellectual answer
4.	What are you feeling now?	*"nothing"* or an intellectual answer
5.	Do you ever get bored?	*"never"*

Example of an intellectual answer:
"No, I'm not angry. That wouldn't be logical."

Anyone who answers all five questions as above is autistic.
Anyone who answers four or fewer as above is not autistic

50 Autistic Traits have a Single Cause

Hyperfocus is the unique and defining characteristic of autism that is responsible for all 50 of its observed traits listed below. Hyperfocus is the perpetual and unrelenting state of intense single-minded concentration fixated on one thought pattern at a time, to the exclusion of everything else. All 50 of these traits are caused by the inability to run two mental programs simultaneously.[1]

Table 2: 50 Autistic Traits Caused by Hyperfocus

Mental Traits	• intense single-mindedness • trapped in thoughts, mind always busy • tends to overthink everything • passionately pursues interests, often to extremes • amasses encyclopedic knowledge about areas of interest • self-awareness but no social awareness • interruptions trigger agitation, confusion, or anxiety • cannot multitask
Sensory Overload	• hypersensitive to loud noises and bright lights • sensory assaults can trigger physiological anxiety • overwhelmed from hearing unwanted conversations • overwhelmed by too much information • sensory overload makes it impossible to think or focus • difficulty conversing or listening to radio while driving
Emotional Traits	• biologically incapable of feeling emotion • incapable of emotionally reacting to anything • processes emotions intellectually • has physiological responses instead of emotions • physiological anxiety warns of unprocessed emotions • incapable of experiencing fear • can be angry without knowing so • never (or rarely) cries or laughs • cannot nurture self psychologically • shrinks from emotional displays by others • unable to defend against emotional attacks
Social Traits	• considers self to be an outsider • lacks innate ability to socialize • unaware of feelings and needs of others • oblivious as to how perceived by others • unaware of socially appropriate responses • cannot pick up on subtleties, unable to take hints
In Conversation	• interested only in information • content of conversation important, context irrelevant

	• speaks factually, without emotion
	• takes everything literally
	• easier to monologue than dialogue
	• misinterprets sarcasm
	• unaware of social cues and nonverbal communication
	• participating in 3-way conversations may be difficult
	• may have difficulty following topic changes
In Relationships	• understands love intellectually but cannot feel love
	• may understand empathy but unable to feel it
	• cannot be emotionally available to others
	• others cannot provide an emotional safety net
Temperament	• drawn more strongly to certain things than to people
	• innate forthrightness tends to scare others
	• never bored, always engaged in mental activity
	• consistent to daily routines; agitated if routine disturbed
	• spontaneity not possible; activities must be pre-planned
	• cannot lie spontaneously; can tell only premeditated lies

Therapy is Harmful

You cannot fix that which is not broken. The autistic brain works in a precise way that cannot be altered.[2] Therapy cannot change neurophysiology.

Applied behavioral analysis (ABA) therapy uses positive reinforcement to help autistic children learn behaviors that are deemed desirable while discouraging undesirable behaviors.[21] There is a vocal community of adults with autism (many of whom had ABA as children) who say that ABA damages mental health and treats them as though they are a problem to be fixed. There is also a higher incidence of PTSD in autistic children who are exposed to ABA.[2]

ABA therapy ignores the child's emotional well-being and quality of life. It assumes that children simply won't do things and need to be incentivized to do them through rewards or lack of rewards. Therapists are unaware that autistic children cannot do what they are being asked to do, or that what they are being asked to do is painful. ABA therapy rewards autistic children to hide their pain and distress.[22]

There are increased symptoms of PTSD in children exposed to ABA therapy.[23] After repeated cycles in the classroom, autistic children begin to develop PTSD because the program focuses on behavior and compliance, and not on what the children are communicating with their behavior.[24]

ABA is based on the cruel premise of trying to make autistic people "normal". Its message is that autistic ways of doing things are wrong and need to be corrected, and that the autistic child is broken and must be molded to be more palatable to non-autistic people. This mistaken belief is destructive of the child's identity and self-worth.[25]

ABA teaches autistic people that their needs are less important than pleasing others. This makes autistic children overly compliant, leaving them vulnerable to manipulation and abuse. These children nee to be taught how to express and get their needs met, not to be taught that their needs are less valid than the needs of people around them.[2]

Differential Diagnosis

Differential diagnosis is distinguishing a specific condition from others that may have similar clinical features. The neurophysiological differences between autism and conditions for which it is mistaken are profound.[26]

Both attention deficit hyperactivity disorder (ADHD) and obsessive-compulsive disorder (OCD) share a common trait, *fickle focus*, which is defined as intervals of intense mental fixation interspersed with episodes of distraction or impulsiveness. Fickle focus can look like hyperfocus that comes and goes; however, true hyperfocus is perpetual and unrelenting. Autistic people never get any relief from hyperfocus.[2]

Because of the confusion between fickle focus and hyperfocus, many people with ADHD or OCD are misdiagnosed as being on the alleged autism spectrum. Also, some who are truly autistic are given false multiple diagnoses that include either ADHD or OCD or both.

Autism is entirely neurophysiological in origin. ADHD and OCD result from neurochemical imbalance. ADHD is caused by low dopamine.[27] OCD is caused by low serotonin.[28]

Table 3: Comparative Neuropsychology

	Autism	**ADHD**	**OCD**
Hyperfocus	Hyperfocus[1]	Fickle focus[2]	Fickle focus[2]
Cingulate Gyrus	Dysfunctional	Functional	Functional
Amygdala	Inactive	Active	Active
Left Frontal Lobe	High alpha activity	High beta activity	High beta activity
Neurochemistry	n/a	Low dopamine	Low serotonin
Concentration	Intense	Intense	intense
Distraction	Never distracted	Sometimes distracted	Self-distracts
Multitasking	Unable to multitask	May multitask	Unable to multitask
Emotional Aspects	Incapable of feeling emotion. Processes emotions intellectually	Can trigger intense emotion	Compulsive behaviors alleviate emotional distress
Social Aspects	Unable to understand and respond to emotional needs of others	Poor social skills	Social anxiety

[1]**Hyperfocus** is perpetual attention fixated on one thought pattern at a time, to the exclusion of all else.
[2]**Fickle focus** is intervals of intense attention interspersed with episodes of distraction or impulsiveness.

Autism versus ADHD

Autism and ADHD are mutually exclusive. You can have one or the other, but not both. People with ADHD tend to be highly emotional. Autistic people are incapable of feeling emotion. Falsely believing autism and ADHD to be alleged co-morbidities is largely responsible for the epidemic of false diagnoses of autism.[19]

Intellectual Guidance System

Autistic people have no innate biologically provided way of experiencing emotions. What they have instead is an intellectual guidance system. They process their emotions intellectually, a process that can take 24 hours, by which time it is too late to have felt anything. Physiological anxiety warns of an unprocessed emotion. Identifying and naming the emotion in question instantly relieves the anxiety.[29]

Conclusions

What makes the autistic brain different is its unique neurophysiology (how it functions). The cingulate gyrus (CG) focuses attention exclusively in the left frontal lobe, creating perpetual and unrelenting hyperfocus, intense single-minded concentration fixated on one thing at a time to the exclusion of everything else.

Autistic people live in a specialized inner space that is entirely intellectual, free from emotional and social distractions. They observe the world in detail without feeling any attachment to what they see. Autistic children come into the world without innate biologically provided ways of emotionally connecting with other people.

Autistic people lack an emotional guidance system. They process their emotions intellectually, a process that can take 24 hours, by which time it is too late to have felt anything. Physiological anxiety warns of an unprocessed emotion. Identifying and naming the emotion in question instantly relieves the anxiety.

Because the amygdala is inactive, autistic people are incapable of experiencing fear. Innate fearlessness makes autistic children vulnerable to dangerous or life-threatening situations. In such situations, autistic adults may feel a mildly heightened sense of awareness while coldly calculating risks and mitigating factors.

References

1. Rowland D. Redefining autism. *Journal of Neurology, Psychiatry and Brain Research* 2020; (02).
2. Rowland D. Autism's true nature. *Journal of Neurology, Psychiatry and Brain Research* 2021; (2).
3. Blatt G. "Autism", *Encyclopedia Britannica*.
4. Montgomery S. *Temple Grandin*. New York, 2012: Houghton Mifflon Harcourt, p 22.
5. Kanner L. "Autistic Disturbances of Affective Contact". *Nervous Child*, 1943.
6. Grandin T, Panek R. *The Autistic Brain*. New York: 2014, First Mariner Books, pp 5-7.
7. Frith, U. *Autism and Asperger Syndrome*. Cambridge, 1991: Cambridge University Press, pp 37-92.
8. Wing L. Asperger syndrome: a clinical account. *Psychological Medicine* 1981; (11):115-129.
9. Bosch G. *Infantile Autism* (trans. D Jordan, I Jordan). New York, 1970: Springer-Vertag.
10. Wing L. Asperger syndrome: a clinical account. *Psychological Medicine* 1981 ;(11):115-129.
11. Rowland D. The neurophysiological cause of autism. *Journal of Neurology & Neurophysiology* 2020; 11(5):001-004.
12. "Autism spectrum disorder (ASD)". *APA Dictionary of Psychology*.
13. "Prevalence of autism spectrum disorder". *Surveillance Summaries*, Centers for Disease Control and Prevention, Dec. 3, 2021. M, Di
14. Elsabbagh M, Divan G, et al. Global prevalence of autism and other pervasive developmental disorders. *Autism Research* 2012; 5:160-179.
15. Rowland D. Epidemic of False Diagnoses of Autism. *Journal of Neurology, Psychiatry and Brain Research* 2023 ; (01).
16. Lundström S, Reichenberg A, et al. Autism phenotype versus registered diagnosis in Swedish children: prevalence trends over 10 years in general population samples. *British Medical Journal* 2015, Apr. 28.
17. Blumberg SJ, Zablotsky B, *et al.* Diagnosis Lost: Differences between children who had and who currently have an autism spectrum diagnosis. *Autism* 2016; (7):783-95.
18. Rodgaard E, Jensen K, *et al.* Temporal changes in effect sizes of studies comparing individuals with and without autism: a meta-analysis. *JAMA Psychiatry* 2019; 76(11):1124-1132.
19. "Are We Overdiagnosing Autism". *Healthline.com*.
20. Basu S, Parry P. The autism spectrum disorder 'epidemic': Need for biopsychosocial formulation.

Australian and New Zealand Journal of Psychiatry 2013; 47(12):1116-8.
21. "All about Applied Behavior Analysis (ABA) Therapy". *PsychCentral.org.*
22. "Why ABA Therapy is Harmful to Autistic People". *AutisticSciencePerson.com*
23. Kupferstein H. Evidence of increased PTSD symptoms in autists exposed to applied behavior analysis. *Advances in Autism* 2018 ;(02).
24. Grant A. Therapist Neurodiversity Collective: *therapistndc.org*
25. "Rebelling Against a Culture that Values Assimilation Over Individuality". *NeurodivergentRebel.com.*
26. Rowland D. Differential diagnosis of autism: a causal analysis. *Journal of Neurology & Neurophysiology* 2020; 11: 489.
27. Wu J, Xiao H, et al. Role of dopamine receptors in ADHD: a systemic meta-analysis. *Mol Neurobiol* 2012; 45(3):605-20.
28. Baumgarten HG, Grizdanovic Z. Role of serotonin in obsessive-compulsive disorder. *Br J Psychiatry Suppl* 1998 ; (35):13-20.
29. Rowland D. Autism as an intellectual lens. *Journal of Neurology, Psychiatry and Brain Research* 2020 ;(01).

Autistic People Biologically Cannot Feel Emotion

© **Rowland D**. Autistic People are Biologically Incapable of Feeling Emotion. *International Journal on Neuropsychology and Behavioural Sciences* 2024;5(1).

> ## Abstract
> Autistic people live in a specialized inner space that is entirely intellectual, free from emotional and social distractions. They observe the world in detail without feeling any emotional attachment to what they see. They have no innate biological way of emotionally connecting with other people. Autistic people process their emotions intellectually, a process that can take 24 hours, by which time it is too late to have felt anything. Because they do not feel emotion, they have no emotional reactions and no emotional memories. All memories are of events that happened about which they felt no emotion at the time and feel no emotion when talking about it afterward.

Introduction

Definition: Autism is perpetual and unrelenting hyperfocus, the state of intense single-minded concentration fixated on one thing at a time to the exclusion of everything else, including one's own emotions. The probable cause of hyperfocus is a dysfunctional cingulate gyrus (CG), that part of the brain which focuses attention.[1]

Description: Autism is an inherent neurophysiological difference in how the brain processes information. Autistic people live in a specialized inner space that is entirely intellectual, free from emotional and social distractions. They observe the world in detail without feeling any emotional attachment to what they see.[1]

Historical Research

Autism, from the Greek word meaning *self*, was coined in 1911 by Swiss psychiatrist, Eugen Bleuler, who used it to describe withdrawal into one's inner world.[2]. Autistic children appear to be in a world of their own, isolated, and alone with senses that can easily overload. These children talk endlessly about one subject, engage in repetitive behaviors (e.g., wringing hands, rocking body), continually repeat certain words or phrases (echolalia), and are resistant to change.[3]

In 1943, psychiatrist Leo Kanner studied the case histories of 11 highly intelligent children who shared a common set of symptoms consistent with autism: the need for solitude, the need for sameness, and to be alone in a world that never varied.[4] Kanner assumed that these children came into the world without innate biologically provid- ed ways of emotionally connecting with other people.[5]

In 1944, medical professor Hans Asperger described "a particularly interesting and highly recognizable type of child" who has an autistic personality that is an "extreme variant of male intelligence." Asperger described four boys who had severe difficulties of social integration that were compensated for by the kind of high level of thought or experience that can lead to exceptional achievements in later life. He chose the label *autism* for this condition as referring to an inherent fundamental disturbance of contact, the shutting off of relations between self and the outside world.[6] Asperger remarked that for those boys, social adaptation has to proceed via the intellect; and in fact they have to learn everything by the intellect. He considered the autistic syndrome to be a stable personality trait that is genetically transmitted in families.[7]

In 1962, psychiatrist Gerhard Bosch compared infantile autism to the Asperger autistic syndrome and considered them to be two variants of the same condition.[8] In 1979, psychiatrist Lorna Wing introduced the term *Asperger syndrome* to describe the autistic personality. Wing personally examined 34 cases fitting Asperger's description of the autism syndrome and found that they had the following 11 traits in common:[9]

- Single-mindedness combined with social isolation,
- Pedantic speech, often consisting of lengthy discourses on favorite subjects,
- Poor comprehension of other people's expressions and gestures,
- Tendency to misinterpret or ignore nonverbal signs,
- Impairment of two-way social interaction,

- Inability to understand rules of social behavior,
- Lack of the intuitive ability to adapt their approaches to fit in with the needs of others,
- Intensely attached to certain possessions,
- Excellent rote memories and intensely interested in one or two subjects,
- Absorb every fact concerning their chosen field and talk about it at length regardless if the listener is interested, and
- Thought processes are confined to a pedantic, literal, and logical chain of reasoning.

Neurophysiology of the Autistic Brain

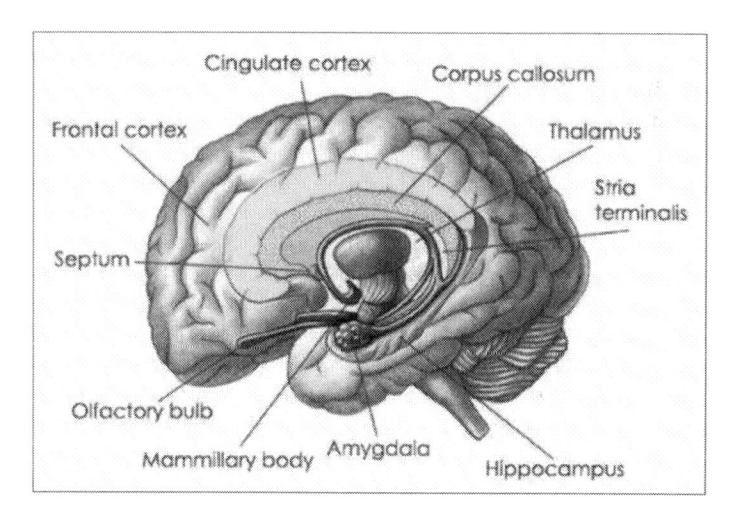

The neurological structure of the autistic brain is the same as for any other brain. What is different about the autistic brain is how it functions with respect to its neurophysiology.

Autistic Neurophysiology

Cingulate Cortex/Gyrus	Dysfunctional	The cingulate gyrus (CG) is that part of the brain which focuses attention. In autism, the CG keeps attention fixated in the left frontal lobe, creating a perpetual state of hyperfocus.
Left Frontal Cortex/Lobe	Dysregulated	In the autistic left frontal lobe, alpha frequencies (8-12 Hz) predominate over beta (12.5-30 Hz), which is the exact opposite of the neurotypical brain. Higher alpha frequencies in the left brain appear to compensate for inability to access creativity and intuition from the right brain.
Right Frontal Cortex/Lobe	Inaccessible	There is normal brainwave activity in the right frontal lobe, with alpha frequencies predominating over beta. However, neural networks may be underdeveloped. The autistic person is completely unaware of anything that happens in the right frontal lobe, the place where emotions and social connectivity are experienced by neurotypical people.
Amygdala	Inactive	The amygdala plays a central role in the expressing of emotions, especially fear. A dysfunctional CG prevents the autistic person from feeling any emotion, with the result that the amygdala is non-functional. An autistic person is incapable of experiencing fear.

In a neurotypical brain, the cingulate gyrus (CG) acts like an automatic transmission that seamlessly switches attention back and forth between frontal lobes, as needed. In autism, a dysfunctional CG keeps the person's attention trapped in the left frontal lobe (logical/analytical) – with no ability to access the right frontal lobe (emotional/creative), which plays a central role in spontaneity, social behavior, and nonverbal abilities. Some neurotypical people are left-brain dominant whereas others are right brain dominant. Autistic people, however, are left brain exclusive. They speak factually, in a monotone voice, and with an expressionless face.[11]

The right frontal lobe, the place where emotions are experienced, is inaccessible to autistic people. The amygdala, the place where emotions are expressed, is inactive in the autistic brain.

These facts are consistent with Leo Kanner's belief that autistic children come into the world without innate biologically provided ways of emotionally connecting with other people.[4]

In a neurotypical brain, the amygdala processes emotions associated with fear and stores emotional memories. When faced with a dangerous situation, the amygdala sounds an alarm that sets off a chain of events: hormones course through the body, pupils dilate, heartrate increases, and the body experiences a "fight or flight" reaction. In extreme situations, all nervous energy goes to the amygdala, which runs totally on instinct and emotion; and that part of the brain that uses logic shuts down completely. In the autistic brain, none of this happens because the amygdala is nonfunctional. In every dangerous situation, the autistic person is fully focused on the event itself and is incapable of feeling fear. Because autistic people do not feel emotion, they have no reaction and no emotional memories. All memories are of events that happened about which they felt no emotion at the time, and about which they feel no emotion when telling someone about it afterward.

Autistic process their emotions intellectually, which process can take 24 hours, by which time it is too late to have felt anything. Physiological anxiety acts as a safety net to warn of any unprocessed emotion. Identifying the emotion in question instantly relieves the anxiety.

Autistic Fearlessness

Autistic people have no involuntary fear response. Innate fearlessness makes autistic children oblivious to danger. In life-threatening situations, the autistic adult is fully focused on the even itself and incapable of feeling fear or even nervousness in that moment. S/he feels a heightened sense of awareness while coldly calculating risks and mitigating factors that quickly form an immediate plan of action. The author of this article is autistic and in his entire life, including 17 years of experience in martial arts, has never once felt fear of any kind.[1] He has never had a fight-or-flight reaction and has no awareness of how that could feel.

Sometimes autistic people may intellectualize about fear, for example saying that after thinking about such-and-such decided it could be a scary thing. However, they are incapable of experiencing any actual fear. If you encounter someone who has never felt fear, this person is most probably locked into autistic hyperfocus.[1]

Litmus Test

Hyperfocus is the unique and defining causal state of autism that creates all of its characteristics. Hyperfocus prevents someone from dividing attention between two thought patterns at the same time. An autistic person talking to you is incapable of feeling any emotion in that moment. The surest way to find out if someone is autistic is to ask these five questions, to which you will receive the following responses:[1]

1.	How often do you cry?	*"never"* or *"rarely"*
2.	How often do you laugh?	*"never"* or *"rarely"*
3.	What are you afraid of?	*"nothing"* or an intellectual answer
4.	What are you feeling now?	*"nothing"* or an intellectual answer
5.	Do you ever get bored?	*"never"*

Example of an intellectual answer: *"No, I'm not angry. That wouldn't be logical."*

Anyone who answers all five questions as above is autistic.
Anyone who answers four or fewer as above is not autistic

50 Autistic Traits Have a Single Cause

Hyperfocus is the unique and defining characteristic of autism that creates all 50 of its observed traits listed below. Hyperfocus is the perpetual and unrelenting state of intense single-minded concentration fixated on one thought pattern at a time, to the exclusion of everything else. All 50 of these traits are caused by the inability to run two mental programs simultaneously.[1]

Mental Traits	• intense single-mindedness • trapped in thoughts, mind always busy • tends to overthink everything • passionately pursues interests, often to extremes • amasses encyclopedic knowledge about areas of interest • self-awareness but no social awareness • interruptions trigger agitation, confusion, or anxiety • cannot multitask
Sensory Overload	• hypersensitive to loud noises and bright lights • sensory assaults can trigger physiological anxiety • overwhelmed from hearing unwanted conversations • overwhelmed by too much information • sensory overload makes it impossible to think or focus • difficulty conversing or listening to radio while driving
Emotional Traits	• biologically incapable of feeling emotion • incapable of emotionally reacting to anything • processes emotions intellectually • has physiological responses instead of emotions • physiological anxiety warns of unprocessed emotions • incapable of experiencing fear • can be angry without knowing so • never (or rarely) cries or laughs • cannot nurture self psychologically • shrinks from emotional displays by others • unable to defend against emotional attacks
Social Traits	• considers self to be an outsider • lacks innate ability to socialize • unaware of feelings and needs of others • oblivious as to how perceived by others • unaware of socially appropriate responses • cannot pick up on subtleties, unable to take hints
In Conversation	• interested only in information • content of conversation important, context irrelevant • speaks factually, without emotion • takes everything literally • easier to monologue than dialogue • misinterprets sarcasm • unaware of social cues and nonverbal communication • participating in 3-way conversations may be difficult • may have difficulty following topic changes
In Relationships	• understands love intellectually but cannot feel love • may understand empathy but unable to feel it

	• cannot be emotionally available to others
	• others cannot provide an emotional safety net
Temperament	• drawn more strongly to certain things than to people
	• innate forthrightness tends to scare others
	• never bored, always engaged in mental activity
	• consistent to daily routines; agitated if routine disturbed
	• spontaneity not possible; activities must be pre-planned
	• cannot lie spontaneously; can tell only premeditated lies

Conclusions

The unique neurophysiology of the autistic brain creates perpetual and unrelenting hyperfocus, a state of intense single-minded concentration fixated on one thing at a time to the exclusion of everything else. Autistic people live in a specialized inner space that is entirely intellectual, free from emotional and social distractions. They observe the world in detail without feeling any emotional attachment to what they see. Autistic children come into the world without innate biologically provided ways of emotionally connecting with other people. Autistic people lack an emotional guidance system. They process their emotions intellectually, a process that can take 24 hours, by which time it is too late to have felt anything. Physiological anxiety warns of an unprocessed emotion. Identifying and naming the emotion in question instantly relieves the anxiety. Because autistic people do not feel emotion, they have no emotional reactions and no emotional memories. All memories are of events that happened about which they felt no emotion at the time and feel no emotion when talking about it afterward.

References

1. Rowland D. Redefining autism. *Journal of Neurology, Psychiatry and Brain Research* 2020;(02).
2. Blatt G. Autism. *Encyclopedia Britannica*.
3. Montgomery S. *Temple Grandin*. New York 2012: Houghton Mifflon-Harcourt, p 22.
4. Kanner L. Autistic disturbances of affective contact. *Nervous Child*.
5. Grandin T, Panek R. *The Autistic Brain*. New York 2014: First Mariner Books, pp 5-7.
6. Frith U. *Autism and Asperger Syndrome*. London 1991:

Cambridge University Press, pp 37-92.
7. Wing L. Asperger syndrome: a clinical account. *Psychological Medicine* 1981;11(1) :115-129.
8. Bosch G. *Infantile Autism* (trans. D. Jordan). New York 1970 : Springer-Vertag.
9. Wing L. Asperger syndrome: a clinical account. *Psychological Medicine* 1981;11(1): 115-129.
10. Rowland D. The neurophysiological cause of autism. *Journal of Neurology & Neurophysiology* 2020:11(5): 001-004
11. Rowland D. Autism as an intellectual lens. *Journal of Neurology, Psychiatry and Brain Research* 2020;(01).

Cholesterol is Irrelevant to Coronary Artery Disease

© **Rowland D**. Free Radicals Cause Coronary Artery Disease; Cholesterol does Not. *OSP Journal of Health Care and Medicine* 2021;2(2).

Abstract

Coronary artery disease is caused by free radical damage to tumor suppressor genes, which mutation allows cells to proliferate out of control to create benign mini tumors between the endothelium lining and the smooth muscle walls of arteries. As these tumors grow, they cause tiny tears in the endothelium that are patched with interlacing filaments of fibrin. This rough scar tissue traps minerals (especially calcium), heavy metals, macrophages, and cellular debris. The final smooth layer of cholesterol that is applied over this arterial plaque plays no causal part in its development. Recent studies indicate that nearly 75 percent of patients hospitalized for a heart attack had cholesterol levels which indicate they were not at high risk for a cardiovascular event, accord- ing to current national cholesterol guidelines. Thus, there is no causal relation between serum cholesterol levels and coronary artery disease.

Background

Heart disease was an uncommon cause of death in the U.S. at the beginning of the 20th century, a time when meat and butter were mainstays of the American diet.[1] Beef, bacon, sausages, and pork were consumed in relatively large quantities. Thus, there is no known causal link between the consumption of cholesterol and the etiology of coronary artery disease.

A national study indicates that nearly 75 percent of patients hospitalized for a heart attack had cholesterol levels that would indicate they were not at high risk for a cardiovascular event, according to current national cholesterol guide- lines.[2] Thus, there is no causal link between serum cholesterol levels and coronary heart disease.

The aim of this study is to determine the true causative agent for coronary artery disease. The methodology used is a critical review of existing literature.

Cholesterol is a Vital Bodily Substance

Cholesterol is a waxy substance that is essential to life. It is a primary component of the membrane that surrounds all human cells. The body uses cholesterol to make hormones (cortisol, estrogen, progesterone, testosterone), to produce vitamin D under the skin in response to sunlight, and to produce bile acids for emulsifying fats for digestion.[3]

Although the brain is only from two to three percent of body weight, 25 percent of bodily cholesterol is found in the brain. In the elderly, the best memory function has been observed in those with the highest level of cholesterol.[4] Low cholesterol is associated with an increased risk for depression and even death.

Cholesterol is so important to health that the liver and intestines produce about 80 percent of it endogenously. Only about 20 percent of bodily cholesterol comes from dietary sources.[5] Vegans, who consume no animal products, produce 100 percent of their bodily cholesterol internally.

The Cholesterol Myth

In 1908 and 1913, Russian researchers fed rabbits diets high in saturated fats and cholesterol.[6,7] Because rabbits are vegetarians, their bodies do not have the enzymes required for metabolizing cholesterol. The blood cholesterol readings in these animals rose to values 10 to 20 times higher than the highest values ever noted in human beings. The entire body of the rabbit becomes overwhelmed with cholesterol that it can neither metabolize, store, nor excrete. It dies not from a heart attack but from starvation. Cholesterol deposits appear in different places in rabbits' blood vessels and have an entirely different structure. There are no hemorrhages, no clefts, and no thrombus formation as there are in human coronary artery disease.[8]

In 1953, Ancel Keys published a report allegedly showing a correlation between the consumption of saturated fats and cholesterol in the incidence of heart disease in six countries.[9] Keys committed selection bias, however, because he had data from 22 countries but chose only those six which supported his foregone conclusion. One of the countries he excluded was France, which has both a high consumption of fat and a low incidence of heart disease. Had Keys plotted all 22 sets of data, there would have been no correlation whatsoever, simply random points on a graph.

A meta-analysis of 26 randomized and controlled cholesterol-lowering trials concluded that there is no significant difference in outcomes from lowering cholesterol, whether by diet or by drugs:[10]

- Fatal heart attacks were the same in treatment and control groups (2.9%);
- Number of deaths was slightly higher in treatment groups (6.1% vs. 5.8%); and
- Number of nonfatal heart attacks was slightly lower in treatment groups (2.8% vs. 3.1%).

Free Radical Hazards

A free radical is a renegade molecule containing an un- paired electron in its outer orbit.[11] The odd number of electrons of a free radical makes it unstable, short lived, and highly reactive. A first free radical instantly pulls an electron from a molecule, thus turning it into a second free radical that begins a chain reaction cascade that finally damages the living cell.[12] Cascading free radicals can alter DNA, creating mutant cells that proliferate out of control causing tumors throughout the body and bulges inside artery walls. Free radical exposure is thus associated with both cancer and coronary artery disease.[12,22]

Exogenous sources of free radicals include environmental pollution, tobacco smoke, industrial solvents, radiation (X-rays, gamma rays), ozone, and chlorinated drinking water and swimming pools.[12] Dietary sources of free radicals include fried foods, polyunsaturated vegetable oils, and nitrite food preservatives.[13-15] Polyunsaturated oils are chemically unstable because they have multiple loose double carbon bonds in their chemical structure. When subject to heat, polyunsaturated molecules oxidize rapidly to form hazardous free radicals.

The intake of polyunsaturated vegetable oils began to increase starting in the early 1900s, at a time when the consumption of butter and lard was on the decline. Unstable linoleic acid, the predominant polyunsaturated fat in vegetable oils, now makes up about 10 percent of total energy intake in the American diet.[14]

Historically, the largest increase in mortality from coronary artery disease parallels increased consumption of unstable polyunsaturated oils. In 1955, stable animal fats became increasingly abandoned in favor of polyunsaturated oils.[34] By 1960, coronary heart disease was killing one in three Americans.[36]

In 1961, polyunsaturated soybean oil became the predominant oil ingredient in processed foods.[35] Mortality from coronary artery disease peaked in the mid-1960s.[36]

The Structure of Arterial Plaque

There is just as much cholesterol circulating through veins as through arteries. However, plaque builds up only in arteries and never in veins. This is further evidence that cholesterol is not a causative factor in coronary artery disease.

Free radicals attack the smooth muscles in artery walls.[16-21,23-25] There are no muscles in veins, which factor makes them immune to free radical attack.

Tumor suppressor genes are proteins that regulate cells during division and replication.[33] When a tumor suppressor gene in an arterial muscle is mutated by free radicals, it allows cells to proliferate out of control thus creating a benign tumor between the endothelium lining and the smooth muscle wall of that artery.

As the tumor grows, tiny tears develop in the endothelium. The first visual evidence of this arterial damage are streaks of foam cells in the arterial wall just beneath the endothelium. Over time these streaks can develop into atherosclerotic plaques, or they can remain stable or even regress.[26]

Foam cells are swollen lipid laden macrophages that have become trapped in rough scar tissue caused by the healing of tiny cuts or tears in the arterial lining.[17,27] When foam cells die, their contents are released and attract more macrophages thus creating an extracellular lipid core near the center to inner surface of each atherosclerotic plaque. The outer, older portions of the plaque become calcified.[28]

When a blood vessel is injured, platelets adhere to each other and the edges of the injury to form a plug that covers the area. This activates the coagulation mechanism by depositing fibrin, a clotting protein. The resulting plug that is formed acts like a scab which retracts to stop the loss of blood.

Fibrin is a whitish protein that is deposited as fine, interlacing filaments containing entangled red and white blood cells and platelets, the whole forming a coagulum or clot.[18] Fibrinogen is the protein in blood plasma that is converted into fibrin by the action of thrombin and in the presence of calcium ions. In other words, fibrin acts like a scab to prevent a cut or tear from bleeding out or hemorrhaging and traps calcium ions before they can form lumps of calcium that would plug arteries and capillaries. This rough scab-like structure on the artery wall becomes a matrix which traps minerals (especially calcium), heavy metals, macrophages, and cellular debris.[29-31] These are all substances that could not possibly adhere to the smooth lining of a healthy artery.

To prevent obstruction from additional debris becoming trapped in the burgeoning atherosclerotic matrix, the body covers it over with a smooth layer of cholesterol. Note that cholesterol is the last substance laid down in the arterial plaque and not the first.

This outer layer of cholesterol tends to become oxidized from further free radical attack.[32] Cholesterol thus appears to serve a dual protective role: (1) to improve blood flow by adding a smooth surface to the damaged arterial wall; and (2) to prevent free radicals from causing further damage to the artery itself.

Conclusion

Coronary artery disease is caused by free radical damage to tumor suppressor genes, which mutation allows cells to proliferate out of control to create benign tumors between the endothelium lining and the smooth muscle walls of arteries. As these mini tumors grow, they cause tiny tears in the endothelium that are patched with interlacing filaments of fibrin. This rough scar tissue traps minerals (especially calcium), heavy metals, macrophages, and cellular debris. The final smooth layer of cholesterol that is applied over this arterial plaque plays no causal part in its development. Statins may reduce excess cholesterol levels; however, they can do nothing for the true cause of coronary artery disease.

References

1. Dalen JE, Alpert et al. The epidemic of the 20th century: Coronary heart disease. *The American Journal of Medicine* 2014; 127(9): 807-812.
2. Fonarow GC, Sachdeva A. (2009) Most heart attack patients' cholesterol levels did not indicate cardiac risk. *American Heart Journal* 2009.
3. "Cholesterol". *Britannica.com*.
4. West R, Beeri MS, et al. (2008). Undefined. *The American Journal of Geriatric Psychiatry* 2008;16(9):781-785.
5. "Managing your cholesterol". *Harvard Special Health Report*, Harvard Medical School.
6. Ignatowski AC Influence of animal food on the organism of rabbits. *S Peterb Izviest Imp Voyenno-Med Akad* 1908;16:154–173.
7. Anitschkow N., Chalatow S. Ueber experiment- elle cholester-insteatose und ihre bedeutung fuer die entstehung einiger pathologischer prozesse. *Zentrbl Allg Pathol Anat* 1913;24:1–9.
8. Ravnskov U (2000) *The Cholesterol Myths*. Washington, DC: 2000, NewTrends Publishing, pp 137-138.
9. Keys A. Atherosclerosis: a problem in newer public health. *Journal of Mount Sinai Hospital* 1953;20:118-139.
10. Ravnskov U. Cholesterol-lowering trials in coronary heart disease; frequency of citation and outcome. *British Medical Journal* 1992;305:15-19.
11. "What are free radicals". *LiveScience.com*.
12. Phaniendra A., Jestadi DB, Periyasamy L. Free radicals: Properties, sources, targets, and their implication in various diseases. *Indian Journal of Clinical Biochemistry* 2014;30(1): 11-

13. Sun Y, Liu, B, et al. Association of fried food consump- tion with all cause, cardiovascular, and cancer mortality: prospective cohort study. *British Medical Journal* 2018, k5420.
14. DiNicolantonio JJ, O'Keefe JH. (2018). Omega-6 vegetable oils as a driver of coronary heart disease: the oxidized linoleic acid hypothesis. *Open Heart* 2018;5(2),e000898.
15. Yoquinto L. "The truth about nitrite in lunch meat". LiveScience.com, 2013.
16. Walia M, Kwan C, Grover AK. Effects of free radicals on coronary artery. *Medical Principles and Practice* 2003;12(1):1-9.
17. "Macrophages". *Taber's Cyclopedic Medical Dictionary (ed 23)* 2017: F.A. Davis Company, pp 1442-1443.
18. "Fibrin". *Taber's Cyclopedic Medical Dictionary* (ed 23) 2017: F.A. Davis Company, p 923.
19. Maxwell, S. Coronary artery disease - free radical damage, antioxidant protection and the role of homocysteine. *Basic Research in Cardiology*, 2000;95(7):I65- I71.
20. Khan F, Butler R. Free radicals in cardiovascular disease. *Proc Royal College Physicians Edinburgh* 1998;28:102-110.
21. Bahoran T, Soobrattee MA. (2006) Free radicals and antioxidants in cardiovascular health and disease. *Internet Journal of Medical Updates* 2006;1(2).
22. Banksonn DD, Kestin M, Rifai V. Role of free radicals in cancer. *Clinics in Laboratory Medicine* 1993;113(2):463-480.
23. Madamanchi NR, Vendrov V, Runge MS. *Arterio- sclerosis, Thrombosis, and Vascular Biology* 2005;25:29-38.
24. Singh R, Devi S, Gollen R. Role of free radicals in atherosclerosis, diabetes and dyslpidaemia: larger- than-life. *Diabetes Metabolism Research and Review* 2015;(2):113-126.
25. Niki E. Do free radicals play causal role in atherosclerosis? Low density lipoprotein oxidation and vitamin E revisited. *Journal of Clinical Biochemistry and Nutrition* 2011;48(1):3-7.
26. "Pathogenesis of Atherosclerosis". *Boston University Medical Center.bu.edu*.
27. "Foam cells". *Wikipedia.org*.
28. Akers AJ, Nicholls SJ, Di Bartolo BA. Plaque calcification. *Arteriosclerosis, Thrombosis, and Vascular Biology* 2019;39(10).
29. Davies MJ. The composition of coronary-artery plaques. *New England Journal of Medicine* 1997;36:1312-1314.
30. Tomey MI, Narula J, Kovacic JC. Advances in the understanding of plaque composition and treatment options: year in review. *Journal of the American College of Cardiology* 2014;63(16):1604-1616.
31. Cebi A, Kaya Y, Gungor H. Trace elements, heavy metals, and vitamin levels in patients with coronary artery disease. *International Journal of Medical Science* 2011;8(6):456-460.

32. Aviram M. Interaction of oxidized low density lipoprotein with macrophages in atherosclerosis, and the antiatherogenicity of of antioxidants. *Eur J Clin Chem Clin Biochem* 1996;34(8):599-608.
33. "Tumor suppressor gene". *Wikipedia.org*.
34. Roccisano D, Kumaratilake JS. Dietary fats and oils: some evolutionary and historical perspectives containing edible lipids for human consumption. *Food and Nutrition Sciences* 2015;07(08):689-702.
35. Blasbalg TL, Hibbela JR. Changes in consumption of omega-3 and omega-6 fatty acids in the United States during the 20th century. *American Journal of Clinical Nutrition* 2011;93(5): 950-962.
36. Jones DS, Greene JA. The decline and rise of coronary heart disease: understanding public health catastrophism. *American Journal of Public Health* 2013;103(7): 1207-1218.

Hypothyroidism: Most Underdiagnosed Disorder

© **Rowland D**. Hypothyroidism: The Underdiagnosed Metabolic Disorder. *OSP Journal of Health Care and Medicine* 2022;3(1)

Abstract

Most cases of hypothyroidism (low thyroid function) go undetected because laboratory tests measure only the presence of thyroid hormone in the blood but cannot tell us how much active hormone reaches the bodily tissues that require it for their metabolism. The main function of the thyroid gland is to regulate metabolism. The primary hormone secreted by the thyroid is thyroxine (T4), which is physiologically inactive. T4 has to be converted into its active form, triiodothyronine (T3), in order to exert its effects. This conversion is catalyzed by the action of deiodinase enzymes that are widely distributed throughout most tissues of the body. If insufficient T3 reaches bodily cells, the result is diminished basal metabolism and concomitant hypothy- roidism. Low thyroid function is a physiological issue that often escapes detection by hormone blood tests. There is, however, a physiological basal temperature test (BTT) that is 100% reliable in detecting hypothyroidism.

Introduction

In the 1930s, physiologist Broda Barnes PhD studied the diverse and debilitating symptoms that resulted from thyroidectomizing baby rabbits. Every cell in their bodies was adversely affected by the lack of thyroid hormone. When thyroid hormone was administered to some of the rabbits, there was quick relief for their multiple problems and a seemingly miraculous return to good health.[6]

When he became a practicing physician, Broda Barnes MD observed the same symptoms as thyroidectomized rabbits in patients whose thyroid blood tests were normal. In the 1970s, Barnes developed a diagnostic test for hypothyroidism known as the basal temperature test (BTT).[1] In his books, Barnes argues that hypothyroidism affects more than 40% of the American population, significantly higher than the prevalence of approximately 5% reported in peer-reviewed medical literature.[2,15]

In 1990, physician Denis Wilson observed that low thyroid symptoms and low body temperatures in the presence of normal thyroid function tests are common due to impaired conversion of thyroxine (T4) to triiodothyronine (T3). Wilson successfully treated these symptoms with sustained-release triiodothyronine (SR-T3).[3]

Body basal temperature measures how efficiently the thyroid gland is functioning, compared to thyroid blood testing which measures only how much hormone is present in the blood but not how active said hormone is. Every metabolic function in the entire body is completely dependent on enzyme function. In turn, enzyme function is highly dependent on bodily temperature. If basal body temperature is below normal, then all enzymes in every cell of the body are under-functioning, thus having a detrimental effect on how efficiently the entire body functions and resulting in many diverse symptoms.[10]

Thyroid Function

The main function of the thyroid gland is to regulate metabolism. Thyroxine (T4) is the primary hormone secreted by the thyroid gland. It has the potential to increase the rate of metabolism of most bodily cells and to affect almost all tissues of the body.[16] Thyroxine itself is physiologically inactive, however. It has to be converted to its active form (T3) before it can exert its effects.[10]

Triiodothyronine (T3) is the physiologically active form of thyroid hormone. Although some T3 is produced by the thyroid gland, most of it is converted from thyroxine (T4) by the action of deiodinase enzymes distributed throughout most tissues of the body.[15] Active thyroid hormone helps to regulate growth, electrolyte balance, oxidative metabolism, differentiation during cell growth, carbohydrate metabolism, protein metabolism, oxygen consumption, the breakdown of fats, and fertility. Deficiencies of either T4 or T3 are associated with drops in metabolic rate and bodily temperature, increases in cholesterol and blood fats, and accumulation of mucoproteins.[10]

Symptoms of Hypothyroidism

Hypothyroidism results from inadequate levels of active thyroid hormone in the body.[5,14] Symptoms of hypothyroidism vary between individuals and tend to develop slowly.[5-11] Commonly noted symptoms include:
- Diminished basal metabolism
- Low body temperature, especially at bed rest
- Muscles stiff in morning, feel need to limber up
- Fail to feel rested, even after sleeping long hours
- Start slowly in morning, gain speed in afternoon
- Gain weight easily, fail to lose on diets
- Increased blood cholesterol level
- Increased sensitivity to cold, prefer warm climates
- Physical sluggishness
- Facial puffiness
- Dry skin
- Dry hair or hair loss
- Poor short-term memory, forgetfulness
- Yellowish tint to skin on palms and soles (carotenemia)
- Constipation
- Menstrual irregularity
- These worse at night: coughing, hoarseness, muscle cramps

Undiagnosed Hypothyroidism

By regulating the rate at which metabolic processes take place, the thyroid gland acts as a gatekeeper. Normal thyroid function protects against disease; low thyroid function allows it easy access. As thyroid activity declines, so does immunity, circulation, and almost every bodily function.[10] Some of the many conditions linked to low thyroid function include benign breast disease, cancer, cellulitis, chronic fatigue, depression, eczema, recurrent headaches, infertility, menstrual irregularities, obesity, premature aging, psoriasis, and rheumatic pain.[11,12]

Hypothyroidism is both rampant and underdiagnosed. The main reason it goes undetected is because doctors rely solely on laboratory tests for making their diagnoses. Unfortunately, most people with hypothyroidism have normal levels of thyroxine (T4) circulating in their blood. Their problem is not that their thyroid glands do not produce enough T4, but rather their bodily tissues do not convert enough of this hormone into its active form (T3) in order to be able to utilize it efficiently.[10,14]

There is no laboratory test that can determine which cells in the body are receiving adequate thyroid hormone and which are not. The most reliable way we have of assessing thyroid function is to measure its effects on body temperature by means of the basal temperature test (BTT).[10]

Inadequate availability of T3 hormone reduces body temperature and thereby adversely affects the rate at which all biochemical processes take place in the body. This is because temperatures above or below the ideal 37^0C (98.6^0F) alter the shape of enzymes (biochemical facilitators), making them a poorer fit for the substrates for which they were designed.[10]

Low levels of T3 reduce body temperature. Low body temperature, in turn, decreases the efficiency at which cells convert T4 into T3, thus putting the body into a conservation mode of reduced capacity. This is a natural form of adaptation in which the body allocates its scarce energy resources only to the most vital functions. Survival becomes the overriding goal. Other activities, such as physical exercise and sex, become a much lower priority.

Basal Temperature Test

The Basal temperature test (BTT) is an accurate self-test for measuring thyroid function. It is far more reliable than any thyroid blood test. This is because the BTT measures the actual result of the most critical thyroid activity, i.e., the maintenance of bodily temperature. Blood tests measure only the amount of thyroid hormone circulating in the blood, which may or may not be typical of how much active hormone (T3) gets to the individual cells that need it.[10,13-15]

Bodily temperature is directly related to thyroid activity. 37°C (98.6°F) is the ideal temperature at which all biochemical reactions function most efficiently. At temperatures below or above this norm, chemical messengers become misshapen and no longer precisely fit the receptor sites they are intended to activate. Basic physics is at work here, namely heat expands and cool contracts. In this case, however, tolerances are very precise. A shift of temperature of a small fraction of a degree can have a significant effect on the degree of fit between enzyme and substrate, neurotransmitter and receptor, hormone and target cell, and anti-body and foreign protein.[10]

The basal temperature test (BTT) requires taking an underarm (axillary) temperature reading first thing in the morning while the body is at complete rest. Men, prepubescent and postmenopausal women can take this test at any time. Menstruating women need to do the BTT on the second and third mornings after their flow starts.[6]

To do the BTT, place an axillary thermometer under the armpit immediately upon awakening and before stirring from bed. Record the reading on two consecutive days. A range of from 36.6°C to 36.8°C (97.8°F to 98.2°F) suggests normal thyroid function. Temperatures below 36.6°C (97.8°F) indicate low thyroid function (hypothyroidism). Temperatures above 36.8°C (98.2°F) suggest an overactive thyroid, unless the person has advanced arthritis that could falsely elevate temperature due to muscular contractions.[6]

An approximation to the BTT can be made by taking oral temperature readings three times per day between the hours of 10 AM and 5 PM. At the end of the day, average these three readings. Average readings below 37°C (98.6°F) suggest hypothyroidism. Readings of 37.3°C (99.1°F) or higher suggest either hypothyroidism, fever caused by infection, or ovulation. Because oral temperatures taken during the day are not strictly related to basal metabolic rate, it is recommended to take oral readings on five consecutive days to rule out extraneous influences.[10]

Administration of Triiodothyronine

Triiodothyronine (T3) is the hormone that regulates basal metabolism. If basal metabolism is low, as indicated by either (a) a basal temperature of less than 36.60C (97.80F), or (b) a consistent daytime temperature of less than 370C (98.60F), then T3 therapy is required.[17]

Triiodothyronine is used in the treatment of hypothyroidism, sometimes in conjunction with thyroxine. Its rapid absorption and short half-life make it more difficult than thyroxine to use in the routine, long-term treatment of hypothyroidism. The starting dose is 20 mcg daily, increasing to a maximum of 60 mcg daily. Unlike thyroxine, which is taken once daily, the larger doses of triiodothyronine are divided into two to three daily doses because of its shorter half-life.[18,19]

Conclusion

Hypothyroidism is the consequence of diminished basal metabolism caused by insufficient active thyroid hormone (triidothyronin, T3) reaching bodily tissues that depend on it for their optimal functioning. Body basal temperature accurately measures the efficiency of thyroid function. If basal temperature is below normal, then all enzymes in every part of the body are under-functioning.

References

1. Barnes B, Galton L. *Hypothyroidism: The Unsuspected Illness.* New York, 1976: Thomas Y. Crowell Company, pp 23-24, 34-50.
2. "Broda Otto Barnes". *Wikipedia.org.*
3. Hollowell JG, Staehling NW. Serum TSH, T(4), and thyroid antibodies in the United States population (1988 to 1984): National Health and Nutrition Examination Survey (NHANES III). *J Clin Endocrinol Metab* 1988;87:489-499.
4. "Wilson's Temperature Syndrome". *Wikipedia.org.*
5. "Hypothyrodism". *The Merck Manual 17th ed* 1999. Whitehouse Station: Merck Research Laboratories, p 94.
6. "Hypothyroidism". *Tabor's Cyclopedic Medical Dictionary 23rd ed* Philadelphia, 2013: F.A. Davis Company.
7. Starr P. *Hypothyroidism.* Springfield, 1954: Charles C. Thomas,

p 46.
8. Thorpe M. 10 Signs and Symptoms of Hypothyroidism. *Healthline.com*.
9. Schwartz MS. *Endocrines, Organs, and their Impact* 3rd ed. New York, 1978.
10. Rowland D. *Endocrine Harmony: The Mind-Body Nutrient Interface*. Seattle, 2018: Amazon.com Inc., pp 23-33.
11. Barnes B, Galton L. *Hypothyroidism: The Unsuspected Illness*. New York, 1976: Thomas Y. Crowell Company, pp 1-16.
12. Means JH, DeGroot LI, Stanbury JB. *The Thyroid and its Diseases*. New York, 1963: McGraw-Hill, pp 321-322.
13. Jackson AS. Hypothyroidism. *Journal of the American Medical Association* 1957;165:121.
14. KImball OP. Clinical hypothyroidism. *Kentucky Medical Journal* 1933;31:488.
15. Wharton GK. Unrecognized hypothyroidism. *Canadian Medical Association Journal* 1939;40:371.
16. "Triiodothyronine". *Tabor's Cyclopedic Medical Dictionary* 23rd ed Philadelphia, 2013: F.A. Davis Company.
17. Akhtar W, Moghal FA. Hypothyroidism and levothyroxine. *Pakistan Journal of Medical and Health Sciences* 2022;16:630-633.
18. Furman BL. *Triiodothyronine xPharm: The Comprehensive Pharmacology Reference, 2007*. Science Direct.com.
19. Furman BL. *Triiodothyronine: Reference Module in Biomedical Sciences*, 2016. Science Direct.com.

DNA is a Binary Computer Program

© **Rowland D**. DNA is a Binary Computer Program of Infinite Possibilities for the Evolution of New Species. *International Journal of Science Academic Research* 2022;03(02): 3471-3474.

Abstract

The objective of this study is to test the hypothesis that comparing DNA encoding to binary computer programming may explain historical evolutionary bursts that go far beyond anything that could have been anticipated by Darwinian natural selection theory. Statistical analysis of biological sequences suggests that randomness may have a negligible effect on evolution. Every organism is preprogrammed with a binary encoded genetic template for what it could evolve to as a species plus endless possibilities for the evolution of new species. Each DNA molecule consists of a base pair of nucleotides, either guanine (G) coupled with cytosine (C), or adenine (A) coupled with thymine (T). GC and AT are base molecules linked together in long chains. This is analogous to binary computer coding in which each molecule is either a "GC" or an "AT" (rather than a "1" or a "0"). Advanced species have significantly less DNA encoding than primitive species. The amphibian that evolved from a fish no longer needs those parts of its DNA that were exclusive to fish and so loses them. Similarly, the lizard loses those parts of its DNA that were required by amphibians, and so on up the evolutionary scale. Every species carries with it disproportionately huge amounts of inactive DNA that they themselves cannot possibly use. This is for the apparent purpose of keeping biological codes in reserve as a backup contingency plan in case of mass extinctions.

Introduction

All living creatures require deoxyribonucleic acid (DNA), the self-replicating genetic material present in their cells as a component of chromosomes. DNA carries elaborate and precisely encoded instructions for cell reproduction.

Each DNA molecule consists of a base pair of nucleotides, either guanine (G) coupled with cytosine (C), or adenine (A) coupled with thymine (T). Human DNA consists of a chain of about three billion of these GC and AT base molecules linked together.

DNA polymerases are enzymes that regulate cellular reproduction by assembling the nucleotide building blocks of DNA.[1] DNA polymerases are highly accurate, with an intrinsic error factor of less than one mistake for every 10^7 nucleotides.[2] This is an error factor of 0.00001 percent. Somehow, our DNA has been programmed with uncanny precision. If only two or three out of 1.5 billion DNA molecules are out of sequence, birth defects or congenital disease can be the result. If only five to 10 of these 1.5 billion molecules are defective, death can be the result.

Binary Programming

GC and AT base molecules linked together in long chains is analogous to binary computer coding. Mechanical computers are programmed in a binary machine language in which each digit is either a "0" or a "1". Living cells are similarly programmed in a binary language in which each molecule is either a "GC" or an "AT". Ten binary codes in sequence make possible $2^{10} = 1,024$ unique combinations. Three billion binary codes in sequence (as in humans) make possible $2^{3,000,000,000}$ unique combinations, which is a number so incredibly huge that it might as well be infinity.

Every life form has its own DNA program. Surprisingly, the simpler the organism, the longer is its DNA chain. The single celled amoeba, for example, has 290 billion nucleotide pairs in its DNA chain, compared to only 2.9 billion pairs in human DNA.[3] The amoeba, however, uses only an infinitesimal fraction of all the DNA that it carries within it.

Why does the simple amoeba have 100 times as many DNA codes as we humans have? For two reasons: (1) every organism carries within its body DNA potential for possible use by subsequently evolved species; and (2) the more evolved a species becomes, the more of its ancestral

DNA is shed as no longer being required. Every living thing carries in its DNA genetic programming for future species to which it could evolve, as an evolutionary reserve. This is proof positive that DNA orchestration has been deliberately planned and could not possibly be the result of random events.

Every species actively uses only a tiny fraction of its DNA. Only about 1.5 percent of human DNA may be active. The other 98.5 percent or so is inactive.[4] Nature must have a reason for continually and consistently reproducing so much inactive DNA in all species. The only plausible explanation is that it provides potential for species to adapt and evolve. Each species comes with a genetic imprint of what it could evolve to as a species, plus endless possibilities for the evolution of new species.

Darwinian evolution presupposes that the development of more advanced life forms can happen only from a combination of these two factors: (1) random mutation, and (2) natural selection. There is a third factor overlooked by evolutionists: (3) cellular adaptation. Cells can acquire new characteristics resulting from interaction with their environment, and these characteristics are inherited by successive generations. In other words, cells can learn and adapt within their own lifetime, making significant changes without having to wait for them to show up in their descendants.

A Deliberate Plan

Evolution is impossible without DNA. Therefore, whatever created DNA also created evolution, and vice versa. Either DNA was the result of random events, or it was orchestrated. There is no third possibility. All the evidence indicates that sophisticated DNA programming could not possibly have been random. DNA binary coding defies evolution.[21]

DNA structure and function are too complex to be explained by known evolutionary mechanisms. The DNA biological system could not have evolved by successive small modifications to pre-existing systems through Darwinian natural selection or random mutation.

Random mutations happen rarely; and most mutations are harmful, making an organism less capable of surviving. Furthermore, DNA copying processes have elaborate built-in repair mechanisms.[22,23] In the rare instances where genetic mutations may be beneficial, they can make only minor changes to organisms and are incapable of developing new body plans. The birth of new species thus requires pre-planning.

It is not possible for programmed DNA to have been the result of random events. In the case of the amoeba, it took foreknowledge (a) to make cytosine combine consistently with thymine, (b) to make adenine combine consistently with guanine, (c) to line up 300 billion of these CT and AG base pairs in an exact binary sequence, (d) to arrange these binary codes with precise logic and nontrivial computing, (e) to create a double helix structure in which an AG purine in one strand always bonds to a CT pyrimidine in another strand, and vice versa, (f) to create self-correcting polymerase enzymes that proofread their work at each stage of DNA development, and (g) to include surgical and chemical ways of correcting DNA damage after the fact.

There is another difficulty with the "DNA just happened" argument. DNA is an essential component of life. Before there was DNA, life did not exist; there were only physical and chemical substances. If the four nucleotides involved in DNA were spontaneously created by means of chemical reactions in multiple locations at various times, how did they seek each other out to form DNA? There is no electromagnetism, no chemical affinity, nor any other physical force drawing them together. Only living organisms are capable of the independent motion required to seek each other out, but nothing was living until there was DNA.

The DNA polymerase enzyme is a protein molecule comprised of over 700 amino acids and requires a template in order to function.[24,25] There is no way that DNA polymerase just happened.

Atrophy of Disuse

Humans, other primates, guinea pigs, and fruit-eating bats suffer from an ancient genetic defect, *hypoascorbemia*, in which the liver has lost its ability to produce L-gulonolactone oxidase, the enzyme which produces vitamin C internally.[5-7] All other mammals produce vitamin C endogenously, which ability gives them immunity to scurvy, viral infections, rheumatoid diseases, cardiovascular conditions, and strokes.

To compensate for its inability to produce vitamin C internally, gorillas must consume 18 to 20 kilograms of vegetation every day (leaves, stems, roots, young branches, buds, bark, piths, seeds, and fruit).[8] This is the equivalent of consuming 4,500 mg. of vitamin C (ascorbic acid) daily from dietary supplements.[6,9]

The only plausible explanation for loss of the ability to produce L-gulonolactone oxidase is that somewhere in the ancient ancestry of these four species, this enzyme was no longer required. They were living in lush vegetation that provided all their requirements for vitamin C from external sources. The DNA molecule that produces L-gulonolactone oxidase atrophied from disuse and could not be passed on to their descendants.

Atrophy from disuse explains why advanced species have significantly less DNA than primitive species. Multicellular fungi no longer need the DNA required to replicate unicellular organisms, and so they lose it. The amphibian that evolved from a fish no longer needs those parts of its DNA that were exclusive to fish and so loses them. Similarly, the lizard loses those parts of its DNA that were required by amphibians ... and so on up the evolutionary scale.

Evolutionary Reserve

We humans have 98.8 percent of our DNA in common with chimpanzees.[10] What makes us different from them is that more of our DNA is active. Chimps may be using only about 70 percent of the same DNA that we are using. The ability of a species to tap into its DNA reserves gives it the potential to take major leaps forward in evolutionary development.

We humans appear to have about 50% of our DNA in common with bananas.[11] This makes sense only if bananas are carrying unused DNA as a contingency plan for the evolution of more advanced species. Little to none of the DNA that bananas have in common with us can possibly be in actual use by them. If it were, one would expect our two species to have at least some physical traits in common. Fruits and primates are as different as two species could possibly be.

Humans and fish diverged from their common ancestor over 450 million years ago, yet nearly 1,000 genes in the pufferfish (*Fugu rubripes*) are identical to previously unidentified ones in humans.[12] Pufferfish use no human DNA. The only reason they can still be carrying it is to provide for the possible evolution of more advanced species.

Primitive species carry forward disproportionately huge amounts of inactive DNA that they themselves will never use. This is for the sole purpose of keeping biological codes in reserve for all possible creatures that could evolve from them. This orchestration provides for limitless development and expansion of existing life forms, thereby providing a backup contingency plan in case of mass extinctions.

Evolution Reboots Itself

About 250 million years ago, there were major volcanic eruptions that continued for some two million years. More than 90 percent of all species were wiped out by this Great Permian Extinction.[13-14] By dipping into its evolutionary reserve DNA, species that survived this extreme global warming eventually evolved into dinosaurs, which dominated the planet for about 165 million years.

About 66 million years ago, a giant asteroid the size of Mt. Everest struck the Earth at a velocity of 45,000 mph.[15-17] It left an impact crater over 100 miles wide that is now buried under the Yucatan Peninsula in Mexico. Over 70 percent of all species, including the dinosaurs, vanished because of this asteroid collision. Those not killed by the impact and its fallout perished because dense clouds of debris blocked the sun, thus halting photosynthesis and starving the life forms dependent upon it. Alligators, crocodiles, frogs, salamanders, and spiders survived; but large land animals did not. Evolution was dealt a serious setback but rebooted, thanks to the inactive DNA potential of the surviving species.

In the next 10 million years following this asteroid disaster, every major animal group that is around today burst onto the scene. There was a prolific divergence of life into new forms and species that had never existed before – including flowering plants, birds, and large mammals (eventually including humans) – all made possible by calling into play unused DNA potential that had been waiting in reserve for just such a contingency. The death of species became the birth of new species.

The only mammals that appear to have existed prior to this asteroid collision were rodents that served as a food source for dinosaurs. It was only after the dinosaurs became extinct that the surviving mammals evolved into more advanced forms, including primates and humans. We owe our existence to the extinction of the dinosaurs.

Mice and humans share about 97.5 percent of their DNA, which amounts to approximately 3.1 billion binary base codes.[18-20] We humans owe our existence to the untapped evolutionary reserve of mice.

If an even greater disaster ever wipes out all life forms except for unicellular organisms, evolution would recreate itself. Amoebae, algae, and fungi contain enough inactive binary DNA coding to create every species that have ever lived or ever could live on Earth.

The Cambrian Explosion

DNA evidence suggests that the first animals started to evolve around 800 million years ago and some 260 million years later there were sponges; varied seafloor creatures shaped like leaves, ribbons, and quilts; algae, flagellates, stromatolite colonies, and worm-like animals. Some of these creatures reproduced sexually.[26,27]

In only the next 11 million years evolution increased dramatically during what is called the *Cambrian Explosion*. This event was characterized by the appearance of many of the major phyla that make up modern animal life.[28-30] Newly developed species included (a) animals with defined heads and tails for directional movement; (b) animals with hard body parts like shells and spines; (c) chordates, animals with a dorsal nerve chord; (d) brachiopods resembling clams; (e) arthropods, the ancestors of spiders, insects, and crustaceans; (f) mollusks; (g) segmented worms; and

(h) species that burrow into the sediments of the seafloor rather than lying on top of it.

During the Cambrian Explosion, the proliferation of new species far outstripped the ability for them to have been created by natural selection. The only explanation for this evolutionary explosion is that animals have built-in abilities to change the expression of their genes by switching on inactive genes and switching off formerly active ones.

A Universal Template

A universal DNA program in which each species accesses only its own sub-module provides unlimited potential for the adaptation of every form of life. This preprogramming ensures that every species carries in its huge reserve of inactive DNA some unused sequences that are common to many other species, both present and future. It makes possible adaptive evolution through the survival of specific genes, rather than the survival of select species. It explains similarities in species that have completely different origins. Two unrelated species can, on separate evolutionary pathways, activate DNA common to both.

Unanswered Questions

There are two questions about traditional evolutionary thinking that beg for answers: (1) How was DNA created, and (2) Why does every organism always pass on to its descendants billions of inactive DNA codes whose only possible purpose can be to serve as untapped potential for new species? Natural selection takes us only as far as understanding how two parents can have offspring with characteristics of both parents, and that the resulting combined DNA may make the children better adapted to their environment than were succeeding generations. However, natural selection is not intuitive. It cannot predict which DNA codes may be required by future generations and future species.

Conclusion

Every organism comes preprogrammed with a binary encoded genetic template for what it could evolve to as a species plus endless possibilities for the evolution of new species. Darwinian natural selection plays only a small and incidental part of this complex evolutionary process.

References

1. Mandal A. "What is DNA Polymerase?" *News Medical.net*.
2. McCulloch SD, Kunkel TA. The fidelity of DNA synthesis by eukaryotic replicative and translesion synthesis polymerases. *Cell Research* 2008;18(1):148-161.
3. *Genome News Network.org*.
4. "Human Genome Project". *Wikipedia.org*.
5. Stone I. Hypoascorbemia, the genetic disease causing the human requirement of exogenous ascorbic acid. *Perspect Biol Med* Autumn 1966;10(1):133-134.
6. Stone I. "The Genetic Disease, Hypoascorbemia, a Fresh Approach to an Ancient Disease and Some of its Medical Implications." *Cambridge University Press* 01 August 2014.
7. "L-gulonolactone oxidase." *Wikipedia.org*.
8. *Gorilla Facts.org*
9. Rowland D. Antioxidant therapy to protect against free radical damage implicated in coronary heart disease and cancer. *OSP Journal of Healthcare and Medicine* 2021;2(2).
10. Ruder K. "Chimp and Human Chromosomes are Compared". *Genome News Network.org*.
11. *Genome News Network.org*.
12. Reinert B. "Pufferfish Genome Reveals Nearly a Thousand Potentially New Human Genes". *Genome News Network.org*.
13. "Siberian Volcanic Eruptions Caused Extinction 205 Million Years Ago, New Evidence Shows". 2017: *ScienceDaily.com*.
14. Rampino MR, Rodriguez S, et al. Global nickel anomaly links Siberian Traps eruptions and the latest Permian mass extinction. *Scientific Reports* 2017;7(1).
15. Smith R. "Here's What Happened the Day the Dinosaurs Died". *National Geographic 2016*; June 11.
16. Black R. "What Happened the Day a Giant, Dinosaur-Killing Asteroid Hit the Earth". *Smithsonian Magazine* 2019; Sept. 9.
17. Kohl S. "A Massive Asteroid Hit Earth 66 Million Years Ago". *Science360.org* 2019; Sept. 15.
18. "Comparing the Mouse and Human Genomes". *NIH Research Matters* 2014; Dec. 8. National Institutes of Health.

19. "Why Mouse Matters". National Human Genome Research Institute.
20. Coghlan A. "Just 2.5% of DNA turns Mice into Men". 2002; May 30. *NewScientist.com*.
21. Tomkins JP. "Three-Dimensional DNA Code Defies Evolution." 2015; April 27. *Institute for Creation Research.org*.
22. Sherwin F. "DNA Paramedics Repair Chromosomes." 2018; July 24. *Institute for Creation Research.org*.
23. Sherwin F. "DNA Repair Research Reveals Astounding Complexity." 2019; August 15. *Institute for Creation Research.org*.
24. "DNA Polymerase". Wikipedia.org.
25. Berg JM, Tymoczko JL, Stryer L. "DNA Polymerases Require a Template and a Primer". *Biochemistry 5th ed.* New York 2020: W H Freeman.
26. Windley BF. "Precambrian". Britannica.com
27. "Early Life on Earth – Animal Origins". National Museum of Natural History.
28. Flannery TF. "Cambrian Explosion." *Britannica.com.*
29. Bagley M. "Cambrian Period: Facts & Information". *Livescience.com.*
30. Bowring SA, Grotzinger JP, et al. Calibrating rates of early Cambrian evolution. *Science* 1993;261(5126): 1293-1298.
31. Wang J, Du PF, et al. VisFeature: a stand-alone program for visualizing and analyzing statistical features of biological sequences. *Bioinformatics* 2020 Feb 15;36(4):1277-1278.

About the Author

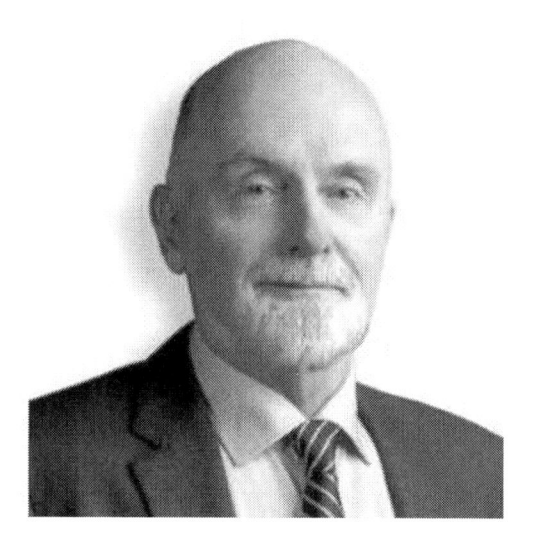

David Rowland

www.davidrowland.name

David Rowland is the prolific author of 83 scientific publications – 47 articles in peer reviewed journals, 16 chapters in medical and scientific research books, plus 20 book editions of his own. David has made contributions to the fields of astrophysics, neuroscience, cardiology, endocrinology, and evolutionary biology. Collectively, David's 47 articles have been read 29,199 times by professors, PhD candidates, and postdoctoral researchers and have been cited 209 times in their research.

Manufactured by Amazon.ca
Bolton, ON